The Hypertension Sourcebook

THE HYPERTENSION SOURCEBOOK

Mary P. McGowan, M.D.
and
Jo McGowan-Chopra

Contemporary Books

Chicago New York San Francisco Lisbon London Madrid Mexico City
Milan New Delhi San Juan Seoul Singapore Sydney Toronto

Library of Congress Cataloging-in-Publication Data

McGowan, Mary P., 1959–
    The hypertension sourcebook / Mary P. McGowan and Jo McGowan-Chopra.
      p.   cm.
    Includes bibliographical references and index.
    ISBN 0-7373-0539-8
    1. Hypertension—Popular works.   I. McGowan Chopra, Jo.   II. Title.

RC685.H8 M34   2001
616.1'32—dc21   00-067785

Contemporary Books

A Division of The **McGraw·Hill** *Companies*

1 2 3 4 5 6 7 8 9 0 DOH/DOH 0 9 8 7 6 5 4 3 2 1

ISBN 0-7373-0539-8

This book was set in Bembo by GTS Graphics
Printed and bound by R. R. Donnelley & Sons Co.

Cover design by Mike Stromberg/The Great American Art Co.
Interior design by GTS Publishing Services

McGraw-Hill books are available at special quantity discounts to use as premiums and sales promotions, or for use in corporate training programs. For more information, please write to the Director of Special Sales, Professional Publishing, McGraw-Hill, Two Penn Plaza, New York, NY 10121-2298. Or contact your local bookstore.

The purpose of this book is to educate. It is sold with the understanding that the publisher and author shall have neither liability nor responsibility for any injury caused or alleged to be caused directly or indirectly by the information contained in this book. While every effort has been made to ensure its accuracy, the book's contents should not be construed as medical advice. Each person's health needs are unique. To obtain recommendations appropriate to your particular situation, please consult a qualified health care provider.

Contents

ॐ

PART III: MANAGING BLOOD PRESSURE IN SPECIAL SITUATIONS

List of Tables

List of Figures and Exhibits

Ȣ

Preface

One year ago I was sitting at our community pool with my sons Patrick and Liam when my cell phone rang. I had expected it to be my husband, Tom, telling me how much longer it would be before he would be leaving the hospital. He had just admitted a fifty-year-old woman who had had a massive stroke. She hadn't seen a doctor in years and by her grief-stricken husband's account, she had terribly high blood pressure but refused to do anything about it. She was on life support, but there was no hope of a recovery. The life support allowed Tom to keep her alive while her family and close friends assembled and processed (or tried to process) the shocking news that a wonderful mother, a best friend, a wife and lover, a dancer, a dreamer was no more. Tom had called me earlier in the day and told me the story. He had never met Mrs. G. before, but as the on-call physician it was his job to admit anyone without a doctor that day. Just before he hung up he had said, "You know, Mary, I really wish I had known Mrs. G. She must have been a wonderful person." I thought later that if he had known her, he would have convinced her to get her blood pressure under control, and she wouldn't be where she was today. He had promised to call me back as soon as he had spoken to everyone in her family, to let me know when to expect him.

When I answered my phone it was Susan Cohen, my literary agent. I told Susan what had been happening. She responded by telling me that high blood pressure was exactly what she wanted to talk to me about. She had just received a call from L. Hudson Perigo, an editor and friend at Lowell House. Hudson was looking for a physician to write a book on hypertension (high blood pressure), and Susan wanted to know if I was interested. My first response was: "Hypertension is not exactly my field (by training I am a cholesterol specialist)." "But don't high blood pressure and high cholesterol go hand and hand?" Susan asked. I had to admit that it was very common for me to see a person for his high cholesterol and proceed to treat both the high cholesterol and high blood pressure. She asked me how many people I had treated for high blood pressure—the answer was literally thousands.

So the "hypertension is not exactly my field" excuse didn't work. Next I asked Susan if she knew that Tom and I were in the process of adopting a baby from Korea. Surely this would stop her from pressing me to do the book. She told me how happy she was for me, but didn't let up. I guess she was thinking I would have time to write on the maternity leave I wasn't anticipating taking.

I tried my last card. "You know I always collaborate with my sister [Jo McGowan Chopra] on any writing project." Jo, a professional writer who lives in India with her husband and three children, had started a school for handicapped children. The school had become a more than full-time job and passion. And on top of the school she had her own writing deadlines. I didn't commit. I told Susan I would talk to Jo and get back to her in a week.

That night I called Jo. She said she would leave the decision up to me, but that she was willing. She even said she thought the project would be fun. I was wavering. Maybe it would be fun, but I also knew if I were going to do it properly, it would require a lot of time. I spoke to the boys, who thought it would be great if Mommy wrote another book with Aunt Jo. Our last book *(Heart Fitness for Life)* meant Jo had made a few extra trips to the United States. Since "Every day is a good day when Aunt Jo is here," the boys were excited at the prospect. I reminded them that it might mean I would have to work a little harder over the next year. "We can do our homework, and you can write your book," was Patrick's suggestion.

When Tom finally got home and the boys were in bed, I mentioned that Susan Cohen had called and asked me if I might be interested in writing a book on hypertension. Tom's response told me I was committed. "Mary, Mrs. G. really could have used a reader-friendly book. If you and Jo can write a book that gets even one person to get her blood pressure under control, then all the work involved will be worth it."

So here it is, *The Hypertension Sourcebook*—written during homework hour for a full year, reworked and improved in India during Jo's children's homework hour. I hope you will find this book a valuable resource. High blood pressure can cause premature heart disease, stroke, kidney failure, and death. But it does not have to. The program outlined in this book will introduce you to lifestyle changes that will dramatically lower your blood pressure. If lifestyle changes alone fail to fully normalize your blood pressure, there are many different medications that lower blood pressure. One will be right for you.

For people with high blood pressure, the future has never looked so good. But it's in your hands. Read this book and decide today to live a long and healthy life.

Acknowledgments

This book would never have come to be had it not been for the extraordinary patience of my husband Tom and children Patrick, Liam, and Sheila. Sheila arrived about halfway through the book and just happened to nap regularly and go to bed early (otherwise the book might never have been completed).

For many people medical school and residency are recalled as a grueling time, with too little sleep and too much intimidation. My experience in medical school and residency was quite the opposite. When I entered medical school at the University of Massachusetts I encountered a group of physicians and teachers whose passion was teaching and whose goal was to make me and my fellow classmates good and caring doctors. The seven years I spent at the University of Massachusetts Medical Center, first as a medical student and later as a resident physician, were challenging, exciting, and yes, exhausting. There was so much to learn and so many people excited to teach. I am especially grateful to Drs. Joseph Alpert, Jim Dalen, Richard Irwin, Lou Braverman, Sarah Cheeseman, David Clive, Mel Pratter, Bruce Weinstein, Nelson Gantz, Abby Adams, Linda Pape, Joel Gore, Ira Ockene, Fran Renzi, and Donna Grogan who taught me not only about illness but about health and motivation. One physician and friend who was an enormous inspiration to me is Sarah Stone. Sarah is one of the most wonderful and caring physicians I have ever met. She was the person who taught me the importance of always remaining a student. She told me that a doctor who has nothing left to learn is a doctor who should retire. That belief stayed with me and made me realize how important it is to continue to ask questions and to question dogma. Sarah helped me realize that the more I know, the more I will be able to teach my patients and that the more I teach the more I learn.

Many people remember the competition and the cutthroat aspects of medical school. At the University of Massachusetts it just did not occur, or at least I did not experience it. I know I learned as much from my classmates as from our teachers. They in turn have become great physicians, teachers, and thinkers. I would like to thank my medical school classmates Drs. John Miller, Anne Cushing-Brescia, Beth Coates, Steven Rapaport, Jim Pellegrini, Seth Bilazarian, Elenie Chadbourne, Andy Coco, Michael Connolly, Elisabeth Haeger, Rawden Evans, Debbie Ehrenthal, Susan Lynch, Caroline Marten-Ellis, Bob Quirbach, Ina Ratner, Mary Ellen Taplin, Dan Sullivan, Kenny Colmer, Dan Carlucci, Kathy Fitzgerald, Ross Carol, Dennis Tighe, Mike Cohen, and Aaron Zuckerberg for their friendship and insights. I would also like to thank my residency colleagues Wayne Hoover, Patty Soscia, Dan Carlucci, Joe Antaki, Denis Dupuis, Grace and Jim Desemone, Renee and Jim Doull, Doug Heller, Bernie Clifford, Martin Boucher, Steve Beaudette, Kristie Silver, Mary Ellen Taplin, Bob McGowen, Adrienne Withers-Bradley, Bob Clinton, David Rind, Sheila Kennedy, Karil Bellah, Michael Thompson, Paul Boffetti, Ron Caputo, Harvey and Allison Goldfine, Larry Greenwald, and Steve Beaudoin for their insights and late-night discussions in the halls of UMass.

As I moved from the University of Massachusetts to Johns Hopkins Hospital, I continued to encounter wonderful teachers and mentors including Drs. Peter Kwiterovich, Stephanie Kafonek, Michele Wilson, and Alain Joffe.

When I left Johns Hopkins I was lucky to take a job at the New England Heart Institute, where our goal is to provide the best possible care to all patients. I would like to thank my partners:

Beatty Hunter, Bob Dewey, Bill Bradley, Pat Lawrence, Connor Haugh, Bruce Hook, Brian Shea, Lou Fink, Michael Hearne, Gary Minkiewicz, Gerry Angoff, Steve Beaudette, Craig Berry, Peter Klemintowicz, Bill Graff, and Mark Liebling for recognizing that preventing a heart attack is as important as performing an angioplasty. The outstanding nurse practitioners and physician's assistants of the New England Heart Institute include: Jeanne Finn, Susan Horton, Judy Tsiorbas, David Allen, Jo-Anne Manson, and Jacqueline Gannuscio.

My colleagues at the Cholesterol Management Center make work a joy. Mary Card, the best dietitian I have ever known, inspires everyone she meets—especially her patients—with her creativity and passion for nutrition and good food; Carolyn Finocchiaro, a gifted and wonderful nurse practitioner, has the perfect combination of gentleness, humor, and authority; Zena Ligon's talent for helping my patients relax makes their blood drawing painless; and Diane Hebert manages my schedule and my life with such dexterity that I move from one thing to another with never a hitch. Thanks also to Elizabeth Schwendler who keeps our hypertension clinical trials on track and to Hope Snazelle, Gail Mullen, and Lisa Klein who make it all happen. I love you all.

Finally I must thank Susan Cohen, my literary agent who suggested I do this project, and Hudson Perigo, an excellent editor who always found a nice way of pushing me along when I was slow in meeting my deadlines.

PART I

HIGH BLOOD PRESSURE —WHAT IS IT?

CHAPTER 1

≈

DO I HAVE IT?

High blood pressure (also called hypertension) is extraordinarily common. The most recent national surveys suggest that fifty million Americans (20 percent of the adult population) have hypertension. By the time Americans reach the age of sixty, six out of ten people have high blood pressure, and it is the second most common reason for a visit to the doctor.

The precise cause of most cases of high blood pressure cannot be determined. In fact, high blood pressure is less likely to be due to one single cause and is typically the result of a complex interaction between an individual's genes and his environment. There is, however, no doubt that certain people are more likely to develop high blood pressure than others. For example, being overweight, having diabetes, and drinking more than two alcoholic beverages per day increase one's risk, especially in those genetically predisposed to hypertension. Certain medications increase the risk. A family history of high blood pressure (especially in your father) means you will be more susceptible yourself. African Americans are at higher risk than are white or Hispanic Americans. And after the age of forty-five, women are at higher risk than men.

Over the past twenty years the National Health and Nutrition Examination Surveys (NHANES) have been conducted three times with the results compiled in reports titled NHANES I, NHANES II, and NHANES III. These surveys are designed to assess the overall health status and dietary habits of the American people. They have evaluated the percentage of people with high blood pressure who are aware of the problem, who have been treated, and whose blood pressure has been reduced to an acceptable level. NHANES III was conducted in two phases, and the results revealed a surprising and disturbing trend (illustrated in Table 1.1).

Table 1.1 High Blood Pressure Awareness, Treatment, and Control in U.S. Adults: 1976–1994

NHANES II (1976–1980)	NHANES III PHASE 1 (1988–1991)	NHANES III PHASE 2 (1991–1994)
Aware of high blood pressure:		
51%	73%	68%
Treated for high blood pressure:		
31%	55%	54%
Controlled to a level below 140/90 mmHg:		
10%	29%	27%

Although it is obvious that great strides have been made during the last twenty years, the trend seen between the first and second phases of the NHANES III survey indicates that among Americans there has been a reduction in awareness, treatment, and control of hypertension. It is frightening to think that only 27 percent of people with high blood pressure are being treated to an acceptable level. The consequences of undertreatment may be deadly. Since high blood pressure predisposes those who have it to heart disease and stroke (our number one and number three causes of death in the United States), failure to treat significantly increases the risk of developing these serious medical conditions. Hypertension is also strongly associated with kidney disease, which frequently progresses so far that dialysis is required.

I hope that by the time you have finished this book, you will have the tools you need to achieve perfect control of your blood pressure, either with lifestyle changes alone (diet, exercise, and supplements) or with lifestyle changes in combination with medications. Although I hope you will find this book valuable and informative, it is not a substitute for working closely with your own personal physician. For example, while exercise is an extremely powerful tool for lowering blood pressure, you should not begin an exercise routine without consulting your doctor. If you have many risk factors for the development of heart disease, suddenly plunging into a demanding new physical routine might do you more harm than good. Your doctor might recommend a stress test to determine if your heart would be compromised by vigorous exercise, and such a test would also help her provide you with guidelines for the duration and intensity of exercise.

Now that we have talked a little about hypertension and how common it is, let's review how blood pressure is measured and help you determine if yours is elevated. And if so, how seriously?

A person's blood pressure is measured using a device called a sphygmomanometer (sfig'-mo-ma-nom-e-ter). A cuff is wrapped around your upper arm and held in place with a Velcro closure. The cuff is then inflated to the point at which your pulse no longer flows in your artery. A stethoscope is placed over the artery at the bend in your arm and the tester listens as the air is gradually released from the cuff and blood forces its way through the artery. A gauge attached to the cuff provides a reading of this maximum amount of pressure, known as the systolic blood pressure. This is the pressure in your arteries when your heart is pumping blood out to your body.

The air continues to be released gradually from the cuff until no sound is heard through the stethoscope. This level represents your diastolic blood pressure or the pressure within your arteries when your heart is relaxed, between heartbeats.

Blood pressure is always expressed as the systolic blood pressure over the diastolic blood pressure, with the systolic figure (representing the peak pressure) always being higher than the diastolic. Blood pressure is measured in millimeters of mercury (mmHg) because the first sphygmomanometers used mercury in the pressure gauge.

The data in Table 1.2 were recently (1997) developed by the Joint National Committee on Prevention, Detection, Evaluation, and Treatment of High Blood Pressure. You can use it to determine where your blood pressure stands.

Table 1.2 Healthy versus High Blood Pressure

CATEGORY	SYSTOLIC BLOOD PRESSURE mmHG		DIASTOLIC BLOOD PRESSURE mmHG
Healthy Blood Pressure			
Optimal	< 120		< 80
Normal	< 130		< 85
High Normal	130–139		85–89
High Blood Pressure			
Stage 1	140–159	and/or	90–99
Stage 2	160–179	and/or	100–109
Stage 3	> 180	and/or	> 110

If you have high blood pressure and you fall into one category for systolic and another for diastolic, you are classified as having the higher stage. For example, a woman with a blood pressure of 150/108 is classified as having Stage 2 hypertension because even though her systolic blood pressure is Stage 1, her diastolic is Stage 2.

High blood pressure needs to be treated, because without therapy a person's risk of developing heart disease and stroke increases dramatically. The absolute risk of developing these conditions is influenced not only by a person's blood pressure but by other risk factors. As you and your doctor make decisions on how best to treat your blood pressure, you will want to take into account your other risk factors. You may want to examine the Coronary Heart Disease (CHD) Score Sheet developed by the investigators from the famous Framingham Heart Study. The Framingham Heart Study examined thousands of men and women in Framingham, Massachusetts, starting more than fifty years ago. The people of Framingham consented to be examined every year or so for decades. Today, many of the offspring of the original Framingham study subjects are study participants themselves. The Framingham study, which did not treat risk factors but rather monitored physical exam findings and blood chemistries, has contributed enormously to our understanding of heart disease. In fact, the study helped prove that smoking, high blood pressure, and high cholesterol were all risk factors for the disease.

You can use the Score Sheets in Table 1.3 to figure out your risk of developing heart disease over the next ten years. There are two different Score Sheets, one for women and one for men. These Score Sheets are only for determining heart disease risk. As far as I know there is no such tool for stroke.

As you can see in Table 1.3, the Score Sheet takes into account age, sex, smoking status, diabetes, and blood pressure in determining risk. In answering the cholesterol section, if you only know your total cholesterol, use the lower chart in step 2; if you know your low-density lipoprotein cholesterol (LDL-cholesterol or bad cholesterol), use the upper chart. Because knowing the LDL-cholesterol is a bit more predictive than just the total cholesterol, go to that column in figuring your points for other risk factors. The only place your point score will differ is under high-density

Table 1.3 CHD Score Sheet for Men

CHD score sheet for men using TC or LDL-C categories. Uses age, TC (or LDL-C), HDL-C, blood pressure, diabetes, and smoking. Estimates risk for CHD over a period of 10 years based on Framingham experience in men 30 to 74 years old at baseline. Average risk estimates are based on typical Framingham subjects, and estimates of idealized risk are based on optimal blood pressure, TC 160 to 199 mg/dL (or LDL-C 100 to 129 mg/dL), HDL-C of 45 mg/dL in men, no diabetes, and no smoking. Use of the LDL-C categories is appropriate when fasting LDL-C measurements are available.

Pts indicates points.

Hard CHID events exclude angina pectoris.

Key Risk

❶	Very low
❷	Low
❸	Moderate
❹	High
❺	Very high

STEP 1 Age

Years	LDL Pts	Chol Pts
30–34	−1	[−1]
35–39	−0	[0]
40–44	1	[1]
45–49	2	[2]
50–54	3	[3]
55–59	4	[4]
60–64	5	[5]
65–69	6	[6]
70–74	7	[7]

STEP 2 LDL-C

Risk	(mg/dL)	(mmol/L)	LDL Pts
❶	<100	<2.59	−3
❷	100–129	2.60–3.36	0
❸	130–159	3.37–4.14	0
❹	160–190	4.15–4.92	1
❺	≥190	≥–4.92	2

[OR] Cholesterol

Risk	(mg/dL)	(mmol/L)	Chol Pts
❶	<160	<4.14	[−3]
❷	160–199	4.15–5.17	[0]
❸	200–239	5.18–6.21	[0]
❹	240–279	6.22–7.24	[1]
❺	≥280	≥7.25	[2]

STEP 3 HDL-C

Risk	(mg/dL)	(mmol/L)	LDL Pts	Chol Pts
❶	<35	<0.90	2	[2]
❷	35–44	0.91–1.16	1	[1]
❸	45–49	1.17–1.29	0	[0]
❹	50–59	1.30–1.55	0	[0]
❺	≥60	≥1.56	−1	[−2]

Reproduced with permission from Wilson PWF et al. *Circulation*. 1998;97:1837–1847.

Table 1.3 CHD Score Sheet for Men, *continued*

STEP 4 Blood Pressure

Risk	Systolic (mm Hg)	<80	80–84	Diastolic (mm Hg) 85–89	90–99	≥100
❶	<120	0 [0] pts				
❷	120–129		0 [0]			
❸	130–139			1 [1]		
❹	140–159				2 [2]	
❺	≤160					3 [3]

STEP 5 Diabetes

Risk		LDL Pts	Chol Pts
❷	No	0	[0]
❸	Yes	4	[4]

STEP 6 Smoker

Risk		LDL Pts	Chol Pts
❷	No	0	[0]
❸	Yes	2	[2]

STEP 7 Adding Up the Points
(sum from steps 1–6)

Age	———
LDL-C or Chol	———
HDL-C	———
Blood Pressure	———
Diabetes	———
Smoker	———
Point total:	———

STEP 8 CHD Risk
(determine CHD risk from point total)

LDL Pts Total	10 Yr CHD Risk	Chol Pts Total	10 Yr CHD Risk
<−3	1%		
−2	2%		
−1	2%	[<−1]	[2%]
0	3%	[0]	[3%]
1	4%	[1]	[3%]
2	4%	[2]	[4%]
3	6%	[3]	[5%]
4	7%	[4]	[7%]
5	9%	[5]	[8%]
6	11%	[6]	[10%]
7	14%	[7]	[13%]
8	18%	[8]	[16%]
9	22%	[9]	[20%]
10	27%	[10]	[25%]
11	33%	[11]	[31%]
12	40%	[12]	[37%]
13	47%	[13]	[45%]
≥14	≥56%	[≥14]	[≥53%]

STEP 9 Comparative Risk
(compare to average person your age)

†Risk estimates were derived from the experience of the Framingham Heart Study, a predominantly Caucasian population in Massachusetts, USA.

‡Low risk was calculated for a person the same age, optimal blood pressure, LDL-C 100–129 mg/dL or cholesterol 160–199 mg/dL, HDL–C 45 mg/dL for men or 55 mg/dL for women, nonsmoker, no diabetes.

Age (years)	Average 10 Yr CHD Risk	Average 10 Yr Hard‡ CHD Risk	Low† 10 Yr CHD Risk
30–34	3%	1%	2%
35–39	5%	4%	3%
40–44	7%	4%	4%
45–49	11%	8%	4%
50–54	14%	10%	6%
55–59	16%	13%	7%
60–64	21%	20%	9%
65–69	25%	22%	11%
70–74	30%	25%	14%

Table 1.3 CHD Score Sheet for Women

CHD score sheet for women using TC or LDL-C categories. Uses age, TC (or LDL-C), HDL-C, blood pressure, diabetes, and smoking. Estimates risk for CHD over a period of 10 years based on Framingham experience in men 30 to 74 years old at baseline. Average risk estimates are based on typical Framingham subjects, and estimates of idealized risk are based on optimal blood pressure, TC 160 to 199 mg/dL (or LDL-C 100 to 129 mg/dL), HDL-C of 55 mg/dL in women, no diabetes, and no smoking. Use of the LDL-C categories is appropriate when fasting LDL-C measurements are available.

Pts indicates points.

Hard CHID events exclude angina pectoris.

Key Risk

❶	Very low
❷	Low
❸	Moderate
❹	High
❺	Very high

STEP 1 Age

Years	LDL Pts	Chol Pts
30–34	−9	[−9]
35–39	−4	[−4]
40–44	0	[0]
45–49	3	[3]
50–54	6	[6]
55–59	7	[7]
60–64	8	[8]
65–69	8	[8]
70–74	8	[8]

STEP 2 LDL-C

Risk	(mg/dL)	(mmol/L)	LDL Pts
❶	<100	<2.59	−2
❷	100–129	2.60–3.36	0
❸	130–159	3.37–4.14	0
❹	160–190	4.15–4.92	2
❺	≥190	≥–4.92	2

[OR] Cholesterol

Risk	(mg/dL)	(mmol/L)	Chol Pts
❶	<4.14	<2.59	[−2]
❷	4.15–5.17	2.60–3.36	[0]
❸	5.18–6.21	3.37–4.14	[0]
❹	6.22–7.24	4.15–4.92	[1]
❺	≥7.25	≥–4.92	[3]

STEP 3 HDL-C

Risk	(mg/dL)	(mmol/L)	LDL Pts	Chol Pts
❶	<35	<0.90	5	[5]
❷	35–44	0.91–1.16	2	[2]
❸	45–49	1.17–1.29	1	[1]
❹	50–59	1.30–1.55	0	[0]
❺	≥60	≥1.56	−2	[−3]

Reproduced with permission from Wilson PWF et al. *Circulation*. 1998;97:1837–1847.

Table 1.3 CHD Score Sheet for Women, *continued*

STEP 4 Blood Pressure

Risk	Systolic (mm Hg)	Diastolic (mm Hg)				
		<80	80–84	85–89	90-99	≥100
❶	<120	−3 [3] pts				
❷	120–129		0 [0]			
❸	130–139			0 [0]		
❹	140–159				2 [2]	
❺	≤160					3 [3]

STEP 5 Diabetes

Risk		LDL Pts	Chol Pts
❷	No	0	[0]
❺	Yes	4	[4]

STEP 6 Smoker

Risk		LDL Pts	Chol Pts
❷	No	0	[0]
❸	Yes	2	[2]

STEP 7 Adding Up the Points
(sum from steps 1–6)

Age	———
LDL-C or Chol	———
HDL-C	———
Blood Pressure	———
Diabetes	———
Smoker	———
Point total:	———

STEP 8 CHD Risk
(determine CHD risk from point total)

LDL Pts Total	10 Yr CHD Risk	Chol Pts Total	10 Yr CHD Risk
<−2	1%	[<−2]	[1%]
−1	2%	[−1]	[2%]
0	2%	[0]	[2%]
1	2%	[1]	[2%]
2	3%	[2]	[3%]
3	3%	[3]	[3%]
4	4%	[4]	[4%]
5	5%	[5]	[4%)
6	6%	[6]	[5%]
7	7%	[7]	[6%]
8	8%	[8]	[7%]
9	9%	[9]	[8%]
10	11%	[10]	[10%]
11	13%	[11]	[11%]
12	15%	[12]	[13%]
13	17%	[13]	[15%]
14	20%	[14]	[18%]
15	24%	[15]	[20%]
16	27%	[16]	[24%]
≥17	≥32%	[≥17]	[≥27]

STEP 9 Comparative Risk
(compare to average person your age)

[†]Risk estimates were derived from the experience of the Framingham Heart Study, a predominantly Caucasian population in Massachusetts, USA.

[‡]Low risk was calculated for a person the same age, optimal blood pressure, LDL-C 100–129 mg/dL or cholesterol 160–199 mg/dL, HDL-C 45 mg/dL for men or 55 mg/dL for women, nonsmoker, no diabetes.

Age (years)	Average 10 Yr CHD Risk	Average 10 Yr Hard[‡] CHD Risk	Low[†] 10 Yr CHD Risk
30–34	<1%	<1%	<1%
35–39	<1%	<1%	1%
40–44	2%	1%	2%
45–49	5%	2%	3%
50–54	8%	3%	5%
55–59	12%	7%	7%
60–64	12%	8%	8%
65–69	13%	8%	8%
70–74	14%	11%	8%

lipoprotein cholesterol (HDL-cholesterol or good cholesterol). If you have an HDL of over 60 mg/dl you get to subtract one point if you are using your LDL and two if you are using total cholesterol.

For example, a fifty-five-year-old man (4 points) who has an LDL-cholesterol of 165 mg/dl (1 point), an HDL-cholesterol of 37 mg/dl (1 point), a blood pressure of 150/100 mmHg (3 points), does not have diabetes (0 points), and is a smoker (2 points) has a score of eleven (4+1+1+3+0+2=11). His ten-year risk of having a heart event such as a heart attack is 33 percent. This is much higher than the 16 percent risk of the average fifty-five-year-old man. This man needs to modify his lifestyle and spelling it out for him in such unambiguous terms is a powerful way to get the message across. I find looking at these Score Sheets very helpful for motivating my patients.

CHAPTER 2

❧

WHAT CAUSES IT? AND WHY SHOULD I WORRY?

Blood pressure is the force required to move blood throughout the body. It makes sense, then, that the determinants of blood pressure are the force generated by the heart as it pumps blood to the body and the resistance or stiffness of the blood vessels themselves.

This sounds simple, but like most things in the human condition, it is anything but. There are literally dozens of situations that can cause problems in either of the primary determinants of blood pressure. Making the situation even more complex is that a given person may have multiple factors that interact and cause hypertension.

What causes high blood pressure? The short answer might look something like this:

1. Too much salt in the diet
2. Kidney disease
3. Stress

4. Aging
5. Overweight
6. Excess alcohol
7. Genetics
8. Certain medications

Some people find this type of list sufficient. In fact, their eyes tend to glaze over if too much scientific detail is presented. For them, the list above can be used to develop a personal program to tackle high blood pressure. Others crave scientific detail. They want to know how cutting back on salt will make a difference to their blood pressure. If you are the first type, skip now to Part II of this book. If you are the second, read on.

SALT INTAKE

One common reason for high blood pressure may be excess sodium (salt) intake. Sodium excess leads to an increase in blood volume. Remember how thirsty you were the last time you ate a salty meal (corned beef, pizza, Chinese food). Salt makes you thirsty, but the extra fluid doesn't just stay in your stomach. It acts to expand your blood volume, which in turn increases blood pressure.

Many people feel that they do not need to worry about salt because their blood pressure is not high (above 140/90 mmHg). The risk of heart disease and stroke doesn't magically begin at this level. In fact, at any level above the optimal blood pressure (below 120/80 mmHg), the risk increases. When Americans with blood pressure readings of 120 to 130 systolic and 80 to 89 diastolic are added to the fifty million with documented high blood pressure, it is evident that 80 percent of Americans over the age of thirty-five are at risk. This is nothing less than an epidemic.

Hypertension experts Drs. Rose and Jeremiah Stamler, a husband and wife team from Northwestern University Medical School in Chicago, have found that systolic blood pressure typically increases by 15 mmHg between the ages of twenty-five and fifty-five. If Americans were to reduce their sodium intake from the average of 4,000 mg per day down to 2,300 mg (or about one teaspoon), blood pressure would still rise, but only by about 6 mmHg. This would result in a 16 percent drop in coronary heart disease deaths and a 23 percent reduction in stroke-related deaths at age fifty-five.

What is the evidence linking sodium with high blood pressure? People from cultures in which salt (often found in processed food) is not part of the diet have much lower blood pressures than do people from societies, like our own, in which salt is abundant and routinely consumed.

The Stamlers helped design and carry out the Intersalt Study, which looked at blood pressure in more than ten thousand men and women ages twenty to fifty-nine worldwide. The more sodium a person was found to have in the urine (urine sodium is a good measure of dietary sodium [salt] intake), the greater the likelihood of finding high blood pressure.

Encouraging studies have shown that infants fed a low-sodium diet had (even fifteen years later), lower blood pressures than did infants fed higher sodium diets. The Stamlers have also shown that simply eating less salt can prevent the development of hypertension (over 140/90 mmHg) in a person with high normal blood pressure (130–139/85–89 mmHg).

Having said that dietary sodium may be responsible for the development of hypertension, it is also important to note that not all people exhibit the same degree of sensitivity to the effects of salt. As a rule, it appears that African Americans and the elderly are less able to handle excess salt in their food. And in the case of salt sensitivity, it seems your mother's response to dietary sodium is the best predictor of your own.

KIDNEY DISEASE

There is no doubt that the kidney is involved in the development of hypertension. People with kidney disease often develop high blood pressure. Given this relationship, it makes sense that low birth weight has been associated with the development of hypertension later in life. Two independent studies (one by Hinchliffe and another by Konje) confirmed that the bulk of kidney development occurs during the last six to eight weeks of pregnancy. The kidneys of premature (low birth weight) babies may therefore fail to develop to the same degree as those of full-term babies. Unfortunately, it appears that this is not correctable even with excellent nutrition after birth. This issue highlights the importance of prenatal care. Many (but obviously not all) premature infants are born to young mothers who fail to seek medical care during pregnancy. Good prenatal care has been clearly demonstrated to decrease the risk of premature birth.

There is also evidence that people with a history of frequent urinary tract infections are at increased risk of developing high blood pressure. People with genetic kidney problems such as polycystic kidney disease almost invariably develop high blood pressure.

The kidney may be involved in the development of high blood pressure in other ways as well (specifically via its role in the production of a chemical called renin). If you have high blood pressure, your doctor may have put you on a medication called an ACE inhibitor (ACE stands for angiotensin–converting enzyme). Examples of ACE inhibitors include:

- Benazepril hydrochloride (Lotensin)
- Captopril (Capoten)
- Enalapril maleate (Vasotec)
- Fosinopril sodium (Monopril)
- Lisinopril (Prinivil, Zestril)
- Moexipril (Univasc)
- Quinapril hydrochloride (Accupril)

- Ramipril (Altace)
- Trandolapril (Mavik)

Or you may be on an AII blocker (angiotensin II receptor blocker). Examples include:

- Losartan potassium (Cozaar)
- Valsartan (Diovan)
- Irbesartan (Avapro)

Your doctor has chosen these medications because he knows that the renin-angiotensin system is involved in the development of high blood pressure. Renin, a chemical found in everybody's blood, is secreted into the blood by the kidney. Renin is responsible for converting another blood chemical called angiotensinogen to angiotensin I. Angiotensin I is, in turn, converted to angiotensin II by the angiotensin-converting enzyme (ACE). Angiotensin II attaches to receptors on the blood vessel, and its presence results in a profound vasoconstriction (clamping down) of the blood vessel. This constriction leads to a dramatic increase in blood pressure. The flowchart in Figure 2.1 tells the story.

Figure 2.1 Kidney Disease and High Blood Pressure

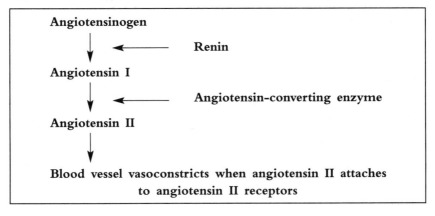

ACE inhibitors prevent the angiotensin-converting enzyme from converting angiotensin I to angiotensin II. Since this prevents angiotensin II from being formed at all, it prevents high blood pressure. Angiotensin II receptor blockers (AII blockers) prevent angiotensin II from attaching to the angiotensin II receptors, which also prevents vasoconstriction of the blood vessels. Many people normalize blood pressure in response to either an ACE inhibitor or an AII blocker. The fact that these drugs work in the treatment of hypertension confirms the importance of the renin-angiotensin system in the development of hypertension. It is likely that in some people a malfunction of this system is the main cause of their high blood pressure.

On the other hand, because there are people in whom these medications lead to no improvement in blood pressure, it is clear that a disturbance in the renin-angiotensin system is not the only cause of hypertension.

STRESS

What about stress? Does stress cause high blood pressure? It appears that it can. When you are under either mental or physical stress, your adrenal gland pumps out epinephrine. You have surely felt the effects of epinephrine before; it is what makes your heart pound and your legs go wobbly when you screech on your car brakes just in time to avoid an accident. Epinephrine, like angiotensin II, is also a vasoconstrictor. Although you might think that the epinephrine released during one single panicky episode of fear would cause no long-lasting effect, there is evidence that the epinephrine released may actually be taken up by nerve endings and then released periodically. So one big scare could be responsible for multiple blood pressure surges. If you have enough large and small stresses over the course of your typical day (children, traffic, arguments), you might end up with sustained high blood pressure.

Does this mean that everyone under stress will develop high blood pressure? Of course the answer is no, but repeated stress over time may lead to high blood pressure in a person genetically susceptible to stress. As far back as 1973, Cobb and Rose documented that air traffic controllers, whose jobs require intense concentration and produce an extraordinary amount of stress, develop high blood pressure at almost six times the rate of people in lower stress jobs.

In 1988, Timio and colleagues noted that cloistered nuns were much less likely to develop high blood pressure than were women of their same age living in the same geographical area but exposed to the stresses of everyday life.

Although there is a substantial body of evidence to suggest that stress can lead to hypertension (possibly through the release of epinephrine, both acutely and chronically), there still remains a great deal of debate about stress in the scientific community. In 1986 Schneider and colleagues found that people who develop hypertension have higher anger and hostility scores than those who do not. They also found these hypertensive people were more likely to suppress their anger. These findings were confirmed by Perini in 1991.

Despite the wealth of data linking stress with the development of hypertension, many scientists still doubt the connection. They point out that stress reduction and meditation, while very important for other reasons, have never been shown to reduce blood pressure. My own belief is that stress, like the other possible precipitants of high blood pressure we have examined in the last few pages, may be the culprit in some but not all people with high blood pressure.

AGING

Still another contributing factor to the development of hypertension is aging. As people age, their arteries become stiffer and the resistance inside them increases, making it more difficult for the heart to pump the blood through. The result is primarily a rise in systolic blood pressure. Isolated systolic hypertension (meaning the diastolic blood pressure remains normal) is very commonly seen in older people, especially women. Interestingly, in societies where people remain very physically active, eat very little salt, and do not gain weight as they age, this increase in arterial stiffness and subsequent high blood pressure does not occur. So aging itself might not be the problem as much as the American pattern of aging.

BEING OVERWEIGHT

Most people know that being overweight is a risk factor for the development of high blood pressure. In fact, in the Framingham Heart Study, approximately 65 percent of the high blood pressure in both men and women was the direct consequence of obesity. In general, for every ten pounds of weight gain Kannel and his colleagues have shown an increase in systolic blood pressure of about 4.5 mmHg. This is a big issue and getting bigger (no pun intended), because approximately 54 percent of the adult population in the United States is either overweight or obese.

Have you stopped to wonder why excess weight leads to high blood pressure? Earlier in this chapter we noted that the primary determinants of blood pressure are cardiac output (the amount of blood pumped out of the heart) and the resistance to the flow of that blood within the body's arteries. People who are obese have a much greater cardiac output than those whose weight is normal; their blood pressure therefore also tends to be higher. It follows, then, that obese people are at higher risk than their normal weight friends of developing heart disease and stroke.

It is not just the high blood pressure that increases an obese person's risk of developing heart disease. Most obese people also have multiple other metabolic abnormalities, but some are at higher risk than others. For example, people who carry most of their weight in the upper body (the so-called apple shape) are at higher risk of heart disease than are people who are obese but carry most of their weight in the lower body (the so-called pear shape). Apple-shaped people are more likely to develop diabetes and high cholesterol levels than pear-shaped people. These added risk factors increase their risk for vascular disease.

Of course it is true that we all know someone (maybe your grandmother) who lived to be ninety-five and was incredibly overweight. Let me assure you, this is the exception, not the rule. How do you know if you are overweight or obese? Weight in pounds is helpful, but the most accurate measure of obesity is body mass index (BMI). The BMI is equal to a person's weight in kilograms divided by his or her height in meters squared. Since it is unlikely you think of your weight in kilograms or your height in meters squared, Table 2.1 will be helpful.

A person is considered overweight if his BMI is 25 or higher and obese with a BMI of 30 or greater. If you are overweight or obese, you can lose weight and keep it off. How much do you need to lose to see major benefits? For many people as little as five to ten pounds will make a big difference. You do not even need to achieve your ideal body weight to dramatically alter your risk of cardiac disease and stroke. One of the most important points I stress again and again in this book is that in order to lose weight and keep it off, you must combine diet with exercise. Almost anyone can lose weight with a diet alone, but almost no one can sustain weight loss without exercise. Recently, Dr C. Everett Koop, the former Surgeon General, went "on-line" to preach this very message. You can visit his Web site at drkoop.com. In truth, you don't want to lower your blood pressure for a month or two; you want to lower it for life. By the time you finish this book you will be armed with a blood pressure–lowering diet and exercise program that will lower your blood pressure for good.

Many obese and overweight people are also insulin resistant. There is a very strong correlation between insulin resistance and the development of hypertension. Insulin is a hormone produced

Table 2.1 Body Mass Index (BMI)★

Weight (lb.)	4'10"	5'0"	5'2"	5'4"	5'6"	5'8"	5'10"	6'0"	6'2"
125	26	24	23	22	20	19	18	17	16
130	27	25	24	22	21	20	19	18	17
135	28	26	25	23	22	21	19	18	17
140	29	27	26	24	23	21	20	19	18
145	30	28	27	25	23	22	21	20	19
150	31	29	27	26	24	23	22	20	19
155	32	30	28	27	25	24	22	21	20
160	34	31	29	28	26	24	23	22	21
165	35	32	30	28	27	25	24	22	21
170	36	33	31	29	28	26	24	23	22
175	37	34	32	30	28	27	25	24	23
180	38	35	33	31	29	27	26	25	23
185	39	36	34	32	30	28	27	25	24
190	40	37	35	33	31	29	27	26	24
195	41	38	36	34	32	30	28	27	25
200	42	39	37	34	32	30	29	27	26
205	43	40	38	35	33	31	29	28	26
210	44	41	38	36	34	32	30	29	27
215	45	42	39	37	35	33	31	29	28
220	46	43	40	38	36	34	32	30	28
225	47	44	41	39	36	34	32	31	29
230	48	45	42	40	37	35	33	31	30

★BMI is defined as body weight (in kg) divided by height (in m^2).

in the pancreas. Its role is to move sugar from the bloodstream into the body's cells. Most adults who develop diabetes started out by being overweight and insulin resistant.

A person is said to be insulin resistant if it takes progressively larger and larger amounts of insulin to move the same amount of sugar into the cells. Ultimately, the pancreas is unable to keep up, the blood sugar level rises, and diabetes develops. Many people who have high blood pressure are found to be insulin resistant, especially if they are also overweight. The connection is so strong that there is a syndrome known as syndrome X or the metabolic syndrome, which consists of high blood pressure, insulin resistance (or diabetes), and elevated blood cholesterol. People with the metabolic syndrome are at very high risk of developing heart disease and stroke.

In obese people, insulin has been found to cause a number of adverse consequences. A major one is sodium (salt) retention (which we have seen can lead to high blood pressure). Another problem is that insulin seems to be able to promote a thickening of the blood vessel walls, which in turn leads to an increase in resistance, resulting in an increase in blood pressure. And while insulin typically causes a blood vessel to dilate (open), in the setting of obesity this does not happen. Finally, insulin may increase the release of hormones like epinephrine, resulting in an increase in blood pressure, as noted earlier in this chapter. As a person loses weight, she often becomes less insulin resistant. This may be one of the ways that weight loss leads to a reduction in blood pressure.

EXCESS ALCOHOL

Excess alcohol is responsible for causing high blood pressure in approximately 10 percent of hypertensive males in the United States. This may come as a surprise to you, given the number of articles promoting alcohol as a way to reduce cardiac risk. It is true that small amounts of alcohol do appear to protect against the development of heart disease (probably through its impact on HDL, the protective cholesterol, and on platelets, our blood-clotting cells). Alcohol raises HDL and seems to impair the function of platelets, thereby decreasing clotting. A reduction in clotting would reduce heart attacks by preventing a clot from forming on a ruptured cholesterol plaque. (This, in fact, is the basis of most heart attacks.) But while alcohol, in small amounts, is probably protective, it appears that at a level greater than two drinks a day for men (less for women), it leads to high blood pressure. One drink is defined as 1.5 ounces of 100-proof liquor, 5 ounces of wine, or 12 ounces of beer. The mechanism by which alcohol causes high blood pressure is not entirely clear. It may be that alcohol alters the cellular transport of calcium, magnesium, and possibly sodium with the end result being high blood pressure. The good news is that if a man who drinks 2 or more ounces of alcohol per day cuts back to just 1 ounce, he can expect a dramatic improvement in his blood pressure. The same is true for women. However, alcohol-related hypertension in women can begin at consumption levels of even 1 ounce per day. Women with high blood pressure should limit alcohol intake to three or fewer drinks a week.

GENETICS

By now it is pretty clear that the road to sustained high blood pressure begins long before your blood pressure is recorded at 140/90 mmHg. It is clear that the interplay of genetics and environmental factors (weight gain, excess alcohol intake, excess salt, and stress) set into motion the cascade that ultimately results in hypertension.

WHO WILL GET HIGH BLOOD PRESSURE?

To some extent it is possible to predict who will develop high blood pressure just by evaluating current blood pressure readings. For example, by using the readings of the participants in the Framingham Heart Study, Kotchen found that over a twenty-six-year follow-up period 24 percent of men and 36 percent of women with initially normal blood pressure went on to develop high blood pressure. This is contrasted with 54 percent of men and 61 percent of women who initially had "high normal" blood pressure. Although the development of high blood pressure was quite high across the board in the participants of this study, it is not hard to see that high blood pressure developed much more commonly in people who initially demonstrated high normal readings. It should come as no surprise, then, that the best predictor of future blood pressure is current blood pressure.

There is no doubt that genetics plays a strong role in predicting who will develop high blood pressure. In families composed of both natural and adopted children, there is a much closer correlation for blood pressure levels between biologic siblings and biologic parent-child pairs than between an adopted child and his non-adopted siblings or parents. Although there is still much to learn, scientists are beginning to find specific gene mutations linked to the condition. There is no doubt that over the next decade, the genetics of high blood pressure will be more clearly defined. This will allow physicians to aim treatment at the specific mutation causing the problem.

MEDICATIONS

Certain medications either cause high blood pressure or interfere with the ability of blood pressure medications to do their job.

In the past, birth control pills were notorious for causing marked increases in blood pressure. Since most women who take birth control pills are now taking pills with a much lower estrogen content, this has become less of an issue. Nonetheless, almost all women who begin the Pill will experience a slight increase in blood pressure. In general this occurs in the setting of a normal or low blood pressure and is not felt to be of any consequence. Currently about 5 percent of women who begin the Pill will develop high blood pressure. Almost invariably these women had "high normal" blood pressure prior to beginning the Pill. Very rarely will a woman who starts on the Pill experience a marked increase in blood pressure. This rare occurrence is very difficult to predict from one's blood pressure readings prior to beginning the medication.

It appears that birth control pill–induced hypertension is caused at least in part by an increase in renin. Remember, an elevated renin level causes an increase in angiotensin II, which is a very powerful vasoconstrictor (meaning it can cause the arteries to clamp down, which increases the pressure within the arteries). Also, women on the Pill may have an expanded blood volume (that is, more blood in the bloodstream). This expanded blood volume, which is caused by the estrogen component of the Pill, increases the blood pressure within the arteries.

When a woman experiences high blood pressure due to the Pill, she should stop its use, or in some cases a pill with a lower dose of estrogen can be used. Some studies have shown that the progestin-only pills or the progestin implants (Norplant) do not cause an unwanted rise in blood pressure. However, progestin-only birth control preparations have an adverse effect on the cholesterol profile. If your doctor suggests a progestin-only form of birth control, make sure to have your cholesterol profile checked prior to starting and three months later.

In almost all situations women who experience high blood pressure while on the Pill will be asked to use another method of birth control. In some situations, however, the risk of pregnancy outweighs the risk of high blood pressure. In such a case the Pill might be continued and a blood pressure medication started. Based on the fact that the high blood pressure associated with birth control pills might be related to an increase in angiotensin (see above), it makes theoretical sense to use drugs that block angiotensin from being formed or from causing the blood vessel to clamp down. Drugs such as Altace, Accupril, Monopril, and Prinivil decrease angiotensin production, and Cozaar, Diovan, Avapro, and Atacand prevent its effect on the blood vessel.

Because of the association between the Pill and the development of high blood pressure, it makes sense that postmenopausal hormone replacement therapy might cause similar problems. But probably owing to the very low doses of hormones that are used, this concern has not been found to be warranted.

Steroids, both oral and high-dose skin creams, can cause high blood pressure. Prednisone, which is often used in the treatment of asthma, has been shown to promote retention of sodium in the bloodstream. When sodium is retained, water is too, resulting in an increase in blood volume, which causes high blood pressure. This same effect is seen when very strong steroid creams are used on the skin. Because steroids can be lifesaving for many conditions, their use is frequently worth the risk of developing high blood pressure. If you require steroids for any reason, it is very important to use the lowest possible dose and have your blood pressure closely monitored.

Many cold medications have warnings on their packages stating that people with high blood pressure should not use them. These cold preparations almost invariably contain one of the following ingredients: ephedrine, pseudoephedrine, phenylephrine, or phenylpropanolamine. These are a family of drugs called sympathomimetic amines, which raises blood pressure by causing vasoconstriction (clamping down). In some cases people who have normal or high normal blood pressure will develop high blood pressure when taking cold remedies. And it is not just the cold pills that can cause this rise in blood pressure; sometimes even the nasal sprays can do it.

It is important to point out that some over-the-counter diet pills contain the same family of sympathomimetic amines. Although you are always better off losing weight on a sensible diet (see chapter 5), if you do buy weight loss pills, read the label carefully and speak to your doctor.

Cyclosporin is a drug given to people who have received an organ transplant (heart, lung, or kidney). This drug is lifesaving because it prevents rejection of the transplanted organ. Unfortunately, it almost uniformly causes an increase in blood pressure. Because of this, an individual taking this drug should have her pressure closely monitored.

People with kidney failure become anemic (low blood count) because their kidneys fail to produce erythropoietin, a hormone that simulates the production of red blood cells. When erythropoietin is given to people with kidney failure, it can boost blood count dramatically and make them feel much more energetic. Unfortunately, up to 35 percent of people taking erythropoietin develop high blood pressure. Many of these people will then require a medication to treat blood pressure.

Nonsteroidal anti-inflammatory drugs (NSAIDs) such as ibuprofen and Naprosyn are commonly used to treat minor aches and pains as well as chronic conditions such as arthritis. These drugs can also cause high blood pressure by promoting salt and water retention. In addition, they also tend to block the ability of most antihypertensives to work. Luckily, the blood pressure–lowering action of the calcium channel blockers (examples: Adalat, Cardizem, and Norvasc) does not seem to be adversely impacted by the NSAIDs.

Gold, which is used in the therapy of some rheumatologic disorders, has also been found to raise blood pressure.

Although it is rare, certain foods can cause high blood pressure. Black licorice, a candy snack, may cause salt and water retention. Licorice is not very popular in the United States, but in Holland, Dubbel Zoote Drops, which are a combination of salt and licorice, are a favorite national sweet. This combination can cause dramatic increases in blood pressure in susceptible people.

Before it was clear that treating high blood pressure reduced the risk of heart attacks, stroke, congestive heart failure, and kidney disease, many studies had a placebo group. From these studies we can determine what happens when high blood pressure is not treated. Between 1967 and 1985, six very large studies were conducted which included more than eleven thousand placebo-treated (thus, untreated) patients. Depending on the degree of blood pressure elevation at the initiation of the study and the follow-up period (which ranged from one to seven years), between 20 and 55 percent of the placebo-treated participants experienced the adverse consequences (heart attack, stroke, kidney disease, congestive heart failure) of high blood pressure. In these trials the people with very, very high blood pressure most commonly experienced stroke, whereas in those with more modest elevations, heart disease was more common.

I

TREATMENT

I hope you are now highly motivated to make lifestyle changes that will lower your blood pressure. Part II of this book will help you develop your own personal program. Once you are found to have high blood pressure, you will need to work closely with your doctor to determine the best therapy. In general you will be asked to work on lifestyle changes for a period of six to twelve months. If these changes fail to control your blood pressure adequately, your doctor will suggest medications. The major exception to this rule is for people who need to get their blood pressure under control quickly. This group of people includes those with very high blood pressure ($\geq 160/\geq 100$) and people with significant coexisting medical conditions such as heart failure, diabetes, or kidney disease. For most people the goal is to achieve a blood pressure of below 140/90. Since 130–139/85–89 is considered high normal, a better goal would be below 130/85. An optimal blood pressure reading is below 120/80.

What can you do to improve your blood pressure? Lots! And you can begin with the following steps:

- Eat a healthy low-fat diet that is high in fruits and vegetables.
- Restrict your intake of sodium (salt).
- Get enough potassium, magnesium, and calcium in your diet.
- Educate yourself regarding which supplements work and which don't.
- Limit your intake of alcohol.
- Lose weight.
- Begin regular exercise.
- Quit smoking.

The following chapters will explore each of these lifestyle changes.

CHAPTER 3

DIET AND BLOOD PRESSURE —THE CRITICAL LINK

The old saying, "You are what you eat" is especially true regarding the development of high blood pressure. Although there is a general consensus that certain aspects of one's diet make it more or less likely that a person will develop high blood pressure, there is considerable debate regarding the relative importance of specific nutrients. At any given age, adults living in industrialized countries have higher blood pressure than do adults living in nonindustrialized societies. As they age, these adults will experience much more substantial increases in blood pressure than will their peers in non-industrialized countries. There is little doubt that diet, exercise, other lifestyle factors, and genetic predisposition all play a role in determining who develops high blood pressure and who does not. This chapter will explore how diet, specific dietary components, dietary supplements, salt, and alcohol influence blood pressure.

As a general rule of thumb, in industrialized societies, vegetarians have lower blood pressure than do people eating a more typical

American diet. And strict vegetarians, for example, those following a macrobiotic diet in which virtually no animal products are consumed, have even lower blood pressure than vegetarians who consume milk and egg products. It would appear, then, that a diet rich in fruits and vegetables might contain certain nutrients that can actually lower blood pressure. It has been hypothesized that potassium and magnesium have a favorable impact on blood pressure. Because of this, clinical trials have been designed to study the influence of potassium and magnesium supplementation.

Likewise, some investigators have reported that a diet rich in calcium resulted in lower blood pressure. This observation naturally prompted a look at the role of calcium supplements as a means of lowering blood pressure. It is also fairly well accepted that a diet rich in heavily processed (high salt) foods will have an adverse effect on blood pressure. Finally, most researchers agree that excess alcohol (more than two ounces per day) adversely affects blood pressure. Reducing alcohol intake can dramatically improve blood pressure in heavy drinkers.

In an attempt to ferret out the impact of fruits and vegetables on blood pressure, the Dietary Approaches to Stop Hypertension (DASH) Trial was designed. The DASH trial was based on the premise that fruits and vegetables and possibly other components of the diet could have a blood pressure–lowering effect. Study investigators recruited 459 middle-aged men and women who had systolic blood pressures less than 160 mmHg and diastolic blood pressures between 80 and 95 mmHg. Approximately 29 percent of the study population had high blood pressure (defined as a systolic blood pressure greater than 140 mmHg, a diastolic blood pressure greater than 90 mmHg, or both) and approximately 60 percent of participants were African Americans.

DASH Trial participants were divided into three groups. Group One (control) ate the typical American diet, low in potassium, high in sodium, and relatively rich in high-fat animal products. Group

Two (combination) consumed a diet high in fruits, vegetables, whole-grain cereals, low-fat dairy products, chicken, fish, and lean meats. In short, in addition to being high in fruits and vegetables, the combination diet was low in fat and cholesterol and high in fiber and minerals. Group Three (fruits and vegetables) ate a diet enriched in fruits and vegetables but otherwise identical to the diet consumed by the control group.

By comparing the blood pressure of people in the combination arm of the study to the blood pressure of those participants following the typical American diet, study investigators were able to evaluate the impact of this diet. By including the fruit and vegetable group, scientists were able to determine how much of the blood pressure–lowering impact of the combination diet could be ascribed to the fruits and vegetables in the combination diet and how much was related to the other aspects of that diet.

Overall the combination diet was found to reduce systolic blood pressure by 5.5 mmHg and diastolic by 3.0 mmHg. The fruit and vegetable diet lowered the systolic and diastolic pressures by 2.8 and 1.1 mmHg, respectively. This might not seem dramatic, but the results were more impressive for the 29 percent of participants who already had high blood pressure. In this group the combination diet resulted in a blood pressure reduction of 11.4/5.5 mmHg (systolic/diastolic). In contrast, participants with high blood pressure who were assigned to the fruit and vegetable diet experienced a drop of 7.2/2.8 mmHg in their systolic and diastolic blood pressures.

In summary, the DASH diet, when followed by people with mild hypertension, can result in about the same degree of blood pressure reduction as a single blood pressure medication. It would appear that the fruit and vegetable component of the diet was responsible for about half of the blood pressure–lowering effect. Since the DASH diet provided participants with whole foods (i.e., fruits, vegetables, whole-grain breads, etc.), it is impossible to know which individual nutrients were responsible for the blood pressure reduction.

Perhaps it is not an individual nutrient alone but a combination of several nutrients consumed together that makes the difference in terms of blood pressure. Nonetheless, it is tempting to speculate that potassium and magnesium are what led to the blood pressure reduction in the fruit and vegetable arm of the study. In the control arm of the DASH Trial, participants consumed about 1,700 mg/day of potassium, whereas in the fruit and vegetable arm, 4,100 mg/day of potassium was consumed.

In order to test the hypothesis that potassium is a critical factor in blood pressure reduction, a series of clinical trials of potassium supplementation have been conducted. Overall, these studies have found that potassium at about 60 mmol/day (this is the normal dose of potassium) resulted in about a 4.4 mmHg drop in systolic and a 2.5 mmHg drop in diastolic blood pressure. Very clearly, then, potassium has a role, but it doesn't explain the entire blood pressure–lowering impact of a diet rich in fruits and vegetables. Interestingly, certain groups of people are more sensitive to potassium supplementation than others. Most affected are people who consume a high salt diet and African Americans.

One other way to increase your potassium intake as you reduce sodium intake is to use salt substitutes. These salt substitutes are extremely high in potassium but contain virtually no sodium. Table 3.1 will help you determine how much potassium the various substitutes are adding to your daily intake.

Table 3.1 Potassium Levels of Salt Substitutes

BRAND	POTASSIUM (MG/TEASPOON)
Morton's	2,465 mg
Adolph's	1,665 mg
Nu-salt	2,025 mg
Diamond Crystal	2,580 mg
No-salt	2,280 mg

What about magnesium supplements? There have been four clinical trials of magnesium supplementation. These trials included from 17 to 461 participants, and the only trial that found any benefit from magnesium supplements was the smallest (17 participants). It is widely believed that the trial was too small to really be predictive, and so it would appear that as a dietary supplement, magnesium has no role in blood pressure reduction.

What about calcium supplements? To be sure, the combination arm of the DASH diet included significant amounts of calcium in the form of low-fat dairy products. Perhaps calcium had a major impact on blood pressure. It may also explain the difference between the blood pressure–lowering impact of the combination diet versus the fruit and vegetable arms of the study.

Pooling the data from multiple clinical trials, we find that calcium supplementation (ranging from 1,000 to 1,500 mg per day) results in about a 1 mmHg drop in systolic blood pressure and no impact on diastolic blood pressure. There are certainly other reasons for calcium supplementation, particularly considering its effect on bone health of older women, but blood pressure reduction does not appear to be one of them.

The combination arm of the DASH diet was, as noted, low in both total and saturated fat. Could this alteration be responsible for some of the blood pressure-lowering impact? Although there is no doubt that blood cholesterol is positively affected by fat restriction, a number of very large studies have found no relationship between fat and blood pressure. However, often people who eat a high-fat diet eat a high-calorie diet. This results in weight gain, which in turn results in high blood pressure.

Fish was also consumed in greater quantities in the combination arm of the DASH diet then in either the control or fruit and vegetable arms. Clinical trials support the role of fish oil supplementation in blood pressure reduction. Unfortunately, the amount of fish oil required to generate any meaningful reduction in blood pressure is so high (on the order of ten to fifteen fish oil capsules per day) that fish oil supplementation is impractical as a treatment of high blood pressure. By the time most people get to three or four fish oil capsules they are complaining of burping a fishy taste, even if they take the fish oil capsules with their evening meal.

In summary, a sensible diet rich in fruits and vegetables, low-fat dairy products, poultry, fish, whole-grain breads and cereals, and low in saturated fat appears the best way to get the nutrients needed to maintain a healthy blood pressure. If you currently consume a diet heavy in processed foods and relatively low in fruits and vegetables—and you have been told that you have high blood pressure—it is likely that eating a diet similar to the one given to participants in the combination arm of the DASH diet will result in as much as an 11 mmHg drop in your systolic blood pressure, and as much as a 5.5 mmHg drop in your diastolic blood pressure. It is important to point out that the DASH diet was specifically designed to keep weight stable. People were asked not to change their exercise habits. If they began to lose weight, extra calories

Table 3.2 DASH Comparison Diets

	SERVINGS PER DAY	
	CONTROL	COMBINATION
Fruit and juice	1.6	5.2
Vegetables	2.0	4.4
Grains	8.2	7.5
Low-fat dairy	0.1	2.0
Nuts, seeds, legumes	0	0.7
Red meats	1.5	0.5
Poultry	0.8	0.6
Fish	0.2	0.5
Fat, oils, and salad dressings	5.8	2.5
Snacks and sweets	4.1	0.7

were provided. In addition, salt restriction was not part of the study. All three study groups consumed about 3,000 mg of sodium per day. So the DASH diet really looked at the impact of dietary changes alone. If your blood pressure is elevated and you switch to a DASH-type diet, lose weight, develop an exercise routine, and cut back on salt, the impact will likely be even more substantial.

As a rule I do not recommend potassium, magnesium, or calcium supplementation for the purposes of blood pressure reduction.

Table 3.2 is a comparison of the control and combination diets expressed as servings per day.

As you try to make your diet look more like the DASH combination diet, it is logical to ask the question: What is a serving? I asked my son (who is six) this same question. His answer: "A serving is how much you eat of something." That is unfortunately exactly what many of my patients think as well. When it comes to serving size, you can use the information in Exhibit 3.1, developed by my colleague, Mary Card, R.D., as a guide.

Exhibit 3.1 Serving Sizes

> Breads, grains, and starches: One serving provides 80 calories and 15 grams of carbohydrate. Examples include:
>
> > 1 cup cold cereal
> > 1 slice bread, 1/2 small bagel, 1/2 English muffin
> > 1/2 cup of pasta, rice, or mashed potatoes
> > 6 crackers, 1 ounce pretzels, 2 rice cakes
> > 1/3 cup cooked beans or lentils
>
> Protein: One serving provides 55 calories, 7 grams of protein, and up to 3 grams of fat. Examples include:
>
> > 1 ounce cooked lean red meat
> > 1 ounce cooked skinless chicken
> > 1 ounce cooked fish
> > 2 ounces shellfish (crab, lobster, shrimp, scallops, clams)
> > 1/4 cup tuna in water

1/4 cup nonfat or low-fat cottage cheese
1/2 cup egg substitute
2 egg whites
1 ounce low-fat cheese (less than 3 grams of fat per serving)
1 ounce (less than 96 percent fat-free luncheon meat)
1/3 cup cooked beans or lentils

Dairy: One serving provides 100 calories and 8 grams of protein. Examples include:

1 cup skim, 1/2%, or 1% milk
1/3 cup dry nonfat milk powder
1 cup plain nonfat yogurt or fruited yogurt sweetened with aspartame

Fruit: One serving provides 60 calories and 15 grams of carbohydrate. Examples include:

1/2 cup fruit juice
1/2 cup canned fruit (packed in water or juice)
1 cup melon (watermelon, honeydew, cantaloupe)
1 cup berries
1/2 banana
1 small apple or orange

Vegetables: One serving provides 25 calories and 3 grams of protein. Examples include:

1/2 cup juice (V-8, tomato, carrot)
1/2 cup cooked vegetables
1 cup raw vegetables

Fats: One serving provides 45 calories and 5 grams of fat. Examples include:

1 tablespoon diet margarine
1 tablespoon light mayonnaise, or light mayonnaise–type salad dressing
1 teaspoon vegetable oil (olive, canola, or peanut oil)
2 tablespoons reduced-calorie salad dressing
1 tablespoon pumpkin or sunflower seeds
2 tablespoons nuts (peanuts, walnuts, filberts, almonds)

Because I suspect you will want to follow the DASH combination diet, I have specifically recommended low-fat products in these serving suggestions.

As I mentioned earlier, the DASH diet did not try to restrict salt, even though salt restriction has clearly been shown to lower blood pressure. The DASH diet held salt constant across each study group to get a clear picture of the impact of other dietary components. You, however, will definitely want to take a look at your salt intake and cut back if necessary. Such a change will likely further improve your blood pressure.

Salt is everywhere. In fact, even people who never pick up the salt shaker eat plenty of it. The National Institutes of Health recommend that all Americans limit their daily intake of salt to 2,400 milligrams. This is equivalent to about 1 teaspoon of table salt. The average American consumes about twice this amount. (The DASH participants actually only consumed 3,000 mg on average.) This is because our diets tend to be rich in processed foods, which are, as a rule, loaded with salt. Since you probably have no plans to move to Borneo or the Fiji Islands, where processed foods are hard to come by, how can you decrease salt in your diet right here at home?

Before moving on, one point of clarification: Salt is really sodium chloride, and sodium makes up 40 percent of sodium chloride. It is the sodium that is responsible for raising blood pressure. When you look at a food label you will notice that sodium is listed. In this book the terms *salt* and *sodium* are being used interchangeably, as they often are in conversation. Just be aware that sodium is the culprit.

The original salt-free diet was the Kempner's rice diet. This diet was popular in the late 1940s when there were next to no medications for the treatment of high blood pressure. The main ingredient of this diet was, you guessed it, rice. The reason a rice diet works to lower blood pressure is that it is very low in sodium. The problem was, the Kempner diet was pretty boring. But a low-sodium diet is not by definition boring, and studies have proven that it doesn't take long for people to adjust their palate so that they desire less salt.

For a lot of people, table salt is not the problem. They take their food as served and never ask for the salt shaker to be passed. But processed and fast foods, which come prepared and which we often believe we have no way of altering, can drive our sodium intake up dramatically.

Reading food labels will help you keep track of the amount of sodium you are getting from processed foods. A word of caution: As you look at food labels, be sure to check what the manufacturer is calling a serving. If you typically consume a cup of something and the manufacturer feels that a serving is half a cup, then you must double everything on the label. For instance, if one-half cup contains 400 milligrams of sodium but you eat a cup, you are taking in 800 milligrams of sodium. I know this sounds pretty obvious, but you would be surprised how many very bright people forget to double calories, fat grams, or sodium as they double the sizes of their portions.

If you are like the average American, you consume about 4,000 to 6,000 milligrams of sodium per day. The ideal way to reduce sodium is by increasing the amount of whole, unprocessed foods you consume. A diet that favors unprocessed foods tends to be rich in fruits and vegetables. Aside from being low in sodium, these foods tend to be high in potassium. And as we have seen, potassium can lower blood pressure in its own right, so reducing sodium while you increase potassium may make a major difference.

I find it helpful to look at a person's typical diet, meal by meal, to determine where the biggest sources of sodium are consumed. It is often the lunchtime selection that does the most damage to sodium levels. For example, a deluxe burger and large fries can add 2,000 milligrams of sodium, not to mention as much as 69 grams of fat (mostly saturated). If you don't go out to lunch, you may find yourself choosing soup, either from a can or a package. This seemingly innocent and often low-fat lunch may contain as much as 600 milligrams of sodium.

Here is a list of tips I give my patients as they aim to reduce sodium in their diets:

1. When possible, always choose the low-salt version of any processed food purchased.
2. Look for the terms "sodium free," "reduced sodium," "less sodium," or "unsalted."
3. Look carefully at the labels of convenience foods. Choose TV dinners with no more than 400 mg of sodium. Look for the low-sodium versions of soups.
4. Avoid fast-food restaurants whenever possible. If you do go to one, choose a grilled chicken sandwich or a salad. If you have a salad, always order your dressing on the side (2 tablespoons of salad dressing generally contain between 210 and 440 milligrams of sodium and about 20 grams of fat). When your dressing arrives in its little cup (it's amazing how much those little cups contain!), don't pour it on; that defeats the purpose. Instead, dip your fork into the dressing and then spear your greens. You coat your fork with the dressing so you get the flavor of the dressing, but you save a great deal on both fat and sodium.
5. Look for the low-sodium versions of all condiments including catsup and soy sauce. (Regular soy sauce has 1,030 milligrams of sodium per tablespoon. Reduced-sodium soy sauce, while better, has a whopping 600 milligrams per tablespoon.)
6. Use salt-free margarine.
7. Buy the low-salt vegetable juices. (Regular tomato juice has a staggering 660 milligrams of sodium in just 6 ounces.)

8. Purchase the low, or, better yet, the no-salt versions of chips, pretzels, crackers, and popcorn.

9. Look at the salt (and fat) content of cheeses. Surprisingly, cottage cheese is loaded with salt; even the low-fat version has about 450 milligrams in a half-cup serving. Other heavy hitters are blue cheese and processed cheese spreads.

10. Beans are an important source of fiber and protein, but the canned varieties tend to be very high in sodium. If you use these for convenience, I suggest that you rinse them several times in cold water, removing about half of the added sodium. Always rinse canned tuna as well.

11. When cooking pasta, rice, or vegetables do not add table salt to the water. Avoid the boxed versions of flavored rice and pasta, as these tend to be very high in sodium.

Get creative with herbs and salt-free seasonings. An excellent publication by the National Heart, Lung and Blood Institute, titled "How to Prevent High Blood Pressure," suggests some ways to "spice up your food" (see Exhibit 3.2).

Exhibit 3.2 Spice Up Your Food

Meat, Poultry, and Fish

Beef: bay leaf, marjoram, nutmeg, onion, pepper, sage, thyme
Lamb: curry powder, garlic, rosemary, mint
Pork: garlic, onion, sage, pepper, oregano
Veal: bay leaf, curry powder, ginger, marjoram, oregano
Chicken: ginger, marjoram, oregano, paprika, poultry seasoning, rosemary, sage, tarragon, thyme
Fish: curry powder, dill, dry mustard, lemon juice, marjoram, paprika, pepper

Vegetables

Carrots: cinnamon, cloves, marjoram, nutmeg, rosemary, sage
Corn: cumin, curry powder, onion, paprika, parsley

Green beans: dill, curry powder, lemon juice, marjoram, oregano,
tarragon, thyme
Greens: onion, pepper
Peas: ginger, marjoram, onion, parsley, sage
Potatoes: dill, garlic, onion, paprika, parsley, sage
Summer squash: cloves, curry powder, marjoram, nutmeg, rosemary,
sage
Winter squash: cinnamon, ginger, nutmeg, onion
Tomatoes: basil, bay leaf, dill, marjoram, onion, oregano, parsley,
pepper

I think you will find the list in Exhibit 3.3 of the sodium content in some common foods and condiments useful.

Exhibit 3.3 Approximate Sodium Content of Common Foods and Condiments

Cereals

Many cereals contain as much as 300 milligrams of sodium, so look closely at your favorite brand.

Cheese

Processed American: 300–460 mg/ounce
Blue cheese: 400 mg/ounce
Brie: 180 mg/ounce
Camembert: 240 mg/ounce
Cheddar: 180 mg/ounce
Colby: 170 mg/ounce
Cottage cheese: 1% fat, 918 mg/cup; 2% fat, 918 mg/cup
Cream cheese: fat free, 160 mg/ounce; low fat, 150 mg/ounce;
regular, 85 mg/ounce
Edam: 275 mg/ounce
Feta: 300 mg/ounce
Goat: hard, 100 mg/ounce; semi-soft, 150 mg/ounce; soft,
100 mg/ounce
Gouda: 230 mg/ounce
Gruyere: 100 mg/ounce
Havarti: 240 mg/ounce

Limburger: 230 mg/ounce
Monterey: 152 mg/ounce
Mozzarella: part skim, 130 mg/ounce; whole milk, 105 mg/ounce
Muenster: 180 mg/ounce
Parmesan: 95 mg/tablespoon
Provolone: 250 mg/ounce
Ricotta: part skim, 150 mg/ounce; whole milk, 100 mg/ounce
Romano: 340 mg/ounce
Swiss: 75 mg/ounce

Condiments, Dressings, and Sauces

Barbecue sauce: 130 mg/tablespoon
Catsup: 100–200 mg/tablespoon
Hollandaise sauce: 600–1,200 mg/packet
Mustard: Grey Poupon, 80 mg/teaspoon; yellow, 65 mg/teaspoon
Pickle slices: bread and butter, 100 mg/2 slices; dill, 140 mg/2 slices
Pickle halves: 325 mg/half
Pickles, whole: 850 mg/3.75 inches long
Relish: 160 mg/tablespoon
Salad dressing: 200–500 mg/2 tablespoons (this degree of variation
    makes it very important to read the label)
Salsa: 200–260 mg/2 tablespoons
Soy sauce: regular, 3,000 mg/1/4 cup; light, 1,900 mg/14 cup
Spaghetti sauce: 400–600 mg/1/2 cup
Steak sauce: 280 mg/tablespoon
Teriyaki sauce: 600 mg/tablespoon

Frozen Meals

Breakfast: Since these meals generally feature some egg/meat
    variation, sodium tends to be high, ranging from 500 to 900
    mg/entree.
Dinner: There is a wide variation, ranging from 450 to 1,200
    mg/entree. Please check the label carefully.

Luncheon Meats

Bologna: 300 mg/ounce
Chicken: 300–400 mg/ounce
Ham: 300–600 mg/ounce
Hot dog: 400–600 mg/hot dog

Roast beef: 400–500 mg/ounce
Salami: 280 mg/ounce
Turkey breast: 300 mg/ounce

Snack Foods

Cheese curls/balls: 380–420 mg/ounce
Corn chips: 170–200 mg/ounce
Popcorn: 5–600 mg/serving (Look closely at the package, the variety,
   and the serving size)
Popcorn/rice/corn cakes: 30–90 mg/cake
Pork skins: 500–700 mg/ounce
Potato chips: 120–350 mg/ounce (Look carefully; some chips are
   much saltier than others)
Pretzels (salted): 490 mg/ounce
Tortilla chips: 150–250 mg/ounce

I hope you don't frequent fast-food restaurants very often. But since it is sometimes unavoidable, the list in Table 3.3 will be helpful in making your selections.

So how much of a reduction in your blood pressure can you expect if you follow a low-sodium diet? It all depends on where your blood pressure was to start with and how salt sensitive you are. Omvik and Myking found a reduction in systolic blood pressure of 8 mmHg and a reduction in diastolic blood pressure of 5 mmHg after six months on a sodium-restricted diet. Most people can begin to see the effect of sodium restriction as early as two weeks into the new diet and the full effect by five weeks. Studies that include people over the age of forty-five or African Americans tend to observe the greatest reductions in blood pressure, because these populations tend to be the most salt sensitive. If you think this degree of blood pressure reduction is minor considering the effort required to lower the salt content of your diet, consider this: Most people don't reduce sodium without increasing potassium, which also lowers blood pressure. And if you are eating more whole foods and less fat, you are likely to lose weight, which again causes

Table 3.3 Calories, Fat, and Sodium in Fast Foods

	CALORIES	FAT (G)	SODIUM (MG)
Boston Market			
Skinless Turkey Breast (5 ounces)	170	1	850
1/4 White Chicken Breast, no skin (4.5 ounces)	210	6	430
Chunky Chicken Salad (3/4 cup)	370	27	800
Original Chicken Pot Pie (15 ounces)	750	34	2,380
Meat Loaf w/Brown Gravy (7 ounces)	390	22	1,040
Ham w/Cinnamon Apples (8 ounces)	350	13	1,750
Steamed Vegetables (2/3 cup)	40	0	40
Herbed Sweet Corn (3/4 cup)	180	4	170
Rice Pilaf (2/3 cup)	180	5	600
Savory Stuffing (3/4 cup)	310	12	1,140
Corn Bread (1)	200	6	390
Oatmeal Raisin Cookie (1)	320	13	260
Cole Slaw (3/4 cup)	280	16	520
Homestyle Mashed Potatoes w/gravy (3/4 cup)	200	9	560
Burger King			
BK Broiler	550	29	480
Hamburger	330	15	530
Jr. Whopper w/Cheese	460	28	770

French Fries (king size)	590	30	1,110
Whopper	630	39	865
Broiled Chicken Salad w/ 2 pkts. Light Italian Dressing	230	11	830
D'Angelo's			
Turkey D'Lite Pokket	330	2	490
Turkey D'Lite Small Sub	365	4	535
Roast Beef D'Lite Pokket	330	6	710
Chicken Stir Fry D'Lite Pokket	360	4.5	1,240
Classic Vegetable D'Lite Pokket	340	10	960
Turkey D'Lite Super Salad	375	4	660
Tuna D'Lite Super Salad	305	2	805
Chicken D'Lite Super Salad	325	4	980
McDonald's			
Hamburger	270	10	530
Cheeseburger	320	14	730
Chicken McNuggets (9)	430	26	870
Quarter Pounder	420	20	690
Big Mac	530	28	960
Chicken Classic (no mayonnaise)	260	4	500

Continued on next page

Table 3.3 continued

Filet O'Fish	360	16	690
French Fries (small)	210	10	135
Grilled Chicken Salad (w/fat-free Herb Vinaigrette)	170	2	570
Chicken Fajita (1)	190	8	310
Grilled Chicken Deluxe (1)	440	20	1,040
Egg McMuffin (1)	290	12	710
Hot Cakes w/syrup & margarine (1 order)	570	16	750
Subway			
Veggie Delite 6"	240	3	590
Roast Beef 6"	300	5	940
Club or Ham 6"	310	5	1,340
Tuna w/Lite Mayonnaise	390	15	940
Tuna Sub 6"	540	32	890
Turkey Club or Ham Salad w/fat-free dressing	180	4	1,230
Chicken or Turkey Sub 6"	320	5	1,190
Pizza (2 slices of 12" pizza)			
Domino's			
Cheese	344	10	981
Veggie	373	12	745

Little Caesar's		
Pepperoni	220	358
Baby Pan	616	1,466
Pizza Hut		
Meat Lovers	501	1,483
Pepperoni Stuffed Crust	460	1,353
Taco Bell		
Bean Burrito	390	1,140
Soft Taco	220	540
Mexican Pizza	570	1,050
Taco Salad w/salsa	840	1,670
Steak Fajita Wrap	460	1,130
Wendy's		
Grilled Chicken Sandwich	310	780
Spicy Chicken Sandwich	410	1,280
Single w/everything	420	810
Chicken Caesar Pita	490	1,300
Garden Veggie Pita	400	780
Garden Ranch Chicken Pita	480	1,170
Chili (small)	190	670

Continued on next page

Table 3.3 continued

Baked Potato	450	<1	450
Broccoli & Cheese Potato	470	14	470
Chili & Cheese Potato	630	24	770
Bacon & Cheese Potato	530	18	1,390
Family-Style Restaurant Items			
Buffalo Wings (12 wings)	700	48	1,750
Stuffed Potato Skins (8 skins)	1,120	79	1,270
Fried Whole Onion (3 cups)	1,690	116	3,040
Sirloin Steak, trimmed (12 ounces)	390	15	470
Filet Mignon, trimmed (9 ounces)	350	18	330
Baked Potato w/1 tablespoon sour cream	280	3	200
Caesar Salad (2 cups)	310	26	620
Chicken Caesar Salad w/dressing (4 cups)	660	46	1,490
Hamburger (10 ounces)	660	36	810
Chicken Chow Mein w/Rice (5 cups)	1,005	32	2,450
Lasagna (2 cups)	960	53	2,060
KFC			
Tender Roast Chicken (1 breast w/o skin)	169	4	797
Original Recipe Chicken (1 breast)	400	24	1,116
Crispy Strips (3 pieces)	261	16	658

Chunky Chicken Pot Pie (1)	770	42	2,160
Original Recipe Chicken Sandwich (1)	497	22	1,213
Cole Slaw (1 order)	180	9	280
Potato Wedges (1 order)	280	13	750
Macaroni & Cheese (1 order)	180	8	860
Arby's			
Hot Ham 'N Cheese (6 1/2" sub)	500	23	1,664
Roast Beef (6 1/2" sub)	700	42	2,034
Breaded Chicken Fillet (1)	536	28	1,016
Roast Chicken Club (1)	546	31	1,103
Light Roast Beef Deluxe (1)	296	10	826
Fish Fillet (1)	529	27	864
French Fries (1 order)	246	13	114
Baked Potato (plain) (1)	355	<1	26
Dairy Queen			
DQ Homestyle Hamburger (1)	290	12	630
DQ Homestyle Cheeseburger (1)	340	17	850
Hot Dog (1)	240	14	730
Chili 'N Cheese Dog (1)	330	21	1,090

an independent reduction in blood pressure. Remember that every little bit counts. Each drop in blood pressure decreases your risk of developing complications such as heart disease, stroke, heart failure, or kidney disease. When you add the blood pressure reduction, the increase in dietary potassium, and weight loss to the reduction achieved with salt restriction, the impact can be dramatic.

The last dietary issue that must be addressed is alcohol. You have probably heard that alcohol reduces the risk of heart disease. Many people ascribe to the philosophy that if a little is good, a lot is better. When it comes to alcohol and heart disease in general and alcohol and blood pressure specifically, this couldn't be further from the truth. It appears that small amounts of alcohol (less than one drink a day for women, less than two drinks a day for men) may reduce the risk of heart disease. In low doses the benefits of alcohol, which include higher HDL-cholesterol (also known as the good cholesterol) level and favorable changes in the blood's ability to clot, win out. At higher levels of intake (greater than a drink a day for women and greater than two drinks a day for men) the negative effects of alcohol predominate. When compared to men, women are less able to handle alcohol because they have much lower levels of gastric alcohol dehydrogenase, the enzyme that metabolizes alcohol.

For the purposes of this book the most important negative effect of alcohol is its impact on high blood pressure. However, it is important to note that women who have more than one drink a day very likely increase their risk of developing breast cancer. Alcohol has been associated with the development of an enlarged and poorly functioning heart, many cancers, liver damage, bleeding in the stomach and elsewhere in the gastrointestinal tract, accidents, suicides, violence, and fetal alcohol syndrome.

If you are a man who typically consumes more than fourteen drinks a week or you are a woman who consumes over seven drinks a week, it is likely that your blood pressure will fall significantly with abstinence or alcohol restriction. In general, the greater the reduction in alcohol intake, the greater the fall in blood pressure.

When people ask me to estimate the amount of benefit they will derive from alcohol restriction, I tell them that for each drink they get rid of, they will likely lower both their systolic and diastolic blood pressures by about 1.3 mmHg each. That might sound trivial, but for some people who cut back by three to four drinks, the change can be quite significant.

It is also very important to point out that in many studies, alcohol intake has been shown to prevent blood pressure medications from doing their job. For some people reducing alcohol intake can make blood pressure medication finally work. Many people also ask: "How long before I see the impact of my alcohol cessation or reduction?" The impact is almost immediate, generally occurring within twenty-four to seventy-two hours.

In summary, lifestyle changes that include adopting a prudent high-fiber, low-fat diet rich in fruits, vegetables, and low-fat dairy products will likely improve your blood pressure. The addition of salt and alcohol restriction may benefit you further. At this point there does not appear to be a role for supplemental vitamins or minerals in blood pressure reduction. Subsequent chapters will explore the role of lifestyle changes on blood pressure. These include exercise, weight loss, and not smoking.

CHAPTER 4

&

DEVELOPING AN EXERCISE PROGRAM

Intuitively we all know that exercise is an important part of a healthy lifestyle. Most people remember a time in their lives when exercise wasn't a chore but a delight. It is hard to know what happened to the person who loved running around the schoolyard playing tag or who was happy to play basketball for hours on end. For most people the transformation is insidious; it begins in high school. If a boy or girl doesn't play on an organized school or town team, daily structured activity generally goes by the wayside. People who do participate in high school athletics typically hang it up at graduation. The fact that the average American gains about a pound a year after completing formal education is directly related to the development of a sedentary lifestyle. Both the reduction in energy expenditure and the weight gain contribute to the age-related rise in blood pressure that is typically seen in industrialized societies.

Countries in which life demands a significant amount of daily physical activity do not experience the marked increase in blood pressure noted in the United States. It is therefore only logical to speculate that an increase in physical activity might prevent the development of high blood pressure and improve levels in those who already have hypertension.

BENEFITS OF EXERCISE

In order to test this hypothesis, more than 45 clinical trials have been conducted. Study subjects have included people with and without high blood pressure. In general, the studies have tested the impact of aerobic activity, but a few have studied the impact of weight training (also known as resistance training). Aerobic means "with oxygen." When you exercise at a steady pace using large muscles, as you do in walking, running, biking, and swimming, you are engaged in aerobic activity. During aerobic exercise your muscles utilize oxygen to burn both glucose (sugar) and body fat. Anaerobic exercise (such as weight training), on the other hand, is performed in short bursts, does not require oxygen, and burns only glucose, not fat. The clinical trials have proven conclusively that regular aerobic exercise lowers blood pressure in both normotensive and hypertensive people. Thankfully, the people who need the greatest reductions (i.e., people who already have high blood pressure) have the greatest response to exercise. Generally speaking, a person with high blood pressure who begins a regular exercise program can anticipate anywhere from a 7 to 10 mmHg drop in systolic blood pressure and about a 5 to 7 mmHg drop in the diastolic reading. For many people this may allow them to avoid medications or at the very least reduce the dose of their blood pressure medications.

Although aerobic and anaerobic activity have both been shown to improve blood pressure and overall cardiovascular health, anaerobic activity can cause a transient increase in blood pressure. For some people the rise can be quite dramatic. For this reason I tend to suggest primarily aerobic activity for my patients who have significant hypertension. However, you may benefit from anaerobic exercise. This is clearly something that needs to be worked out between you and your personal physician. In fact, before you begin any exercise routine, aerobic or anaerobic, I urge you to consult your personal physician, who knows your case best. If you choose anaerobic exercise, I strongly recommend that it be added to your aerobic program (as opposed to replacing it).

Be aware that even an aerobic activity can become anaerobic if you push too hard. If you are markedly short of breath and unable to talk during exercise, you have likely switched to anaerobic metabolism. Burning muscles, which suggests a buildup of lactic acid, is another clue that you may have switched to anaerobic metabolism.

As you embark on an exercise program, it is important to ask: What do I want this program to do for me? To be sure, if you are reading this book you probably want your exercise program to lower your blood pressure. Many people with high blood pressure also need to lose weight, and you may be hoping that an exercise program will help you in this regard as well. It is important to be clear regarding your expectations from an exercise program, for the amount of time and effort you must devote to it differs according to your goals.

Say you are lean and you have no need to lose weight, but you still have high blood pressure. You want to know: What is the least amount of time I can exercise and still get cardiovascular benefit and blood pressure reduction? The short answer is three days a week, 30 minutes per session (more in a moment regarding intensity).

Alternatively, say you would like to lose 20 pounds. You know this will require dietary changes, but you are hoping your exercise program will not only lower your blood pressure but will promote weight loss as well. You want to know: What is the least amount of time I can exercise and still lose weight, lower my blood pressure, and improve my cardiovascular fitness? The short answer here is six to seven days a week, 45 to 60 minutes per session. The main difference here is the need to lose weight. Anyone can lose weight with a diet, but no one can *maintain* that loss without exercise. And it can't be just a whiff of exercise. It needs to be the equivalent of walking 20 miles a week. In our program we tend to favor walking because it has a very low injury rate. Moreover, walking requires no special skills or equipment; it can be done year round, alone or with friends; and it can easily be incorporated into your daily routine.

As you plan your exercise program it is important to keep three things in mind: frequency, intensity, and time (also known as the F. I.T. principle).

Exercise Frequency

Ultimately how frequently you exercise will depend on your fitness goals. If you have never exercised before, it is important to start off slowly. Even if your goal is weight loss, exercising only three times a week gets you started and achieves a conditioning effect, but prevents burnout. If weight loss is your goal, you will ultimately need to double the frequency to a minimum of six times a week.

Exercise Intensity

To make the most of your exercise program it is important to work at the proper intensity. Intensity means how hard you are pushing yourself. You want to be working hard enough to achieve a training effect, that is, turn fat into muscle, but not so hard that you kick your body into anaerobic metabolism.

How can you tell if you are exercising at the proper intensity? One way is by checking your pulse and determining your target heart rate. You can check your pulse in any number of locations:

- your neck, the carotid pulse
- your wrist, the radial pulse
- behind your knee, the popliteal pulse
- on your foot, the dorsal pedis pulse

Each beat of your heart creates a pulse that you can feel and count, and one of the easiest places to check your pulse is at your wrist. Place your index and middle fingers on the thumb side of your wrist. Here you will feel your radial pulse. Count the number of pulses over a 10-second period and multiply this number by 6 to get your pulse rate per minute. Your heart rate (the number of times your heart beats per minute) is an indirect measurement of how hard you are exercising. The target heart rate (THR) range is a common method of measuring exercise intensity.

First figure your maximum heart rate using the following formula:

220 − your age = maximum heart rate (MHR)

Example: A fifty-year-old male or female:

220 − 50 = 170 beats per minute

In order to lower your blood pressure and achieve physical fitness, it is not necessary to work out at your maximum heart rate. In fact, this would be undesirable, especially as you begin a regular exercise program. Studies have determined that exercising at between 50 and 85 percent of your maximum heart rate is sufficient to produce excellent results and a training effect. Again, using the same fifty-year-old man or woman to determine the THR, use the following equations:

170 × 0.50 = 85 beats per minute

170 × 0.85 = 145 beats per minute

The THR range is therefore 85 to 145 beats per minute Table 4.1 will help you determine your own target heart rate and 10-second pulse.

Some people have a great deal of difficulty measuring their pulse. Others are on blood pressure medications that slow their heart rate. Beta-blockers, for example, generally drop the pulse to

Table 4.1 Target Heart Rates

AGE	MAXIMUM HR	TARGET HR	10-SECOND PULSE
20	200	100–170	17–28
25	195	98–166	17–28
30	190	95–162	16–27
35	185	92–157	16–27
40	180	90–153	15–26
45	175	88–149	15–26
50	170	85–145	14–25
55	165	82–140	14–25
60	160	80–136	13–24
65	155	78–131	13–24
70	150	75–128	12–23
75	145	72–123	12–23
80	140	70–119	11–22

60 beats per minute or less, so people on these medications may find it impossible to achieve their target heart rate with exercise. This does not mean this group of people should not exercise or if they do, that they will not be able to accurately assess the intensity of their programs. The "Talk Test" is by far the easiest (and fairly accurate) method of determining whether you are exercising at the appropriate intensity to achieve aerobic fitness. As its name implies, as you are exercising you should be able to talk without huffing and puffing excessively. However, you should be slightly winded, enough so that delivering the Gettysberg Address would not be possible. If you can do that, you need to push a little harder.

Time
The issue of time has already been partially addressed. Clearly you want to spend enough time on your exercise program to achieve

cardiovascular fitness and to reduce your blood pressure. The bare minimum is 30 minutes three times a week (this does not include warm-up and cool-down times). But for most of my patients who are hoping for weight loss, this is not enough. People desiring weight loss must generally spend 45 to 60 minutes per day if they choose an exercise like walking and about 30 minutes per day if they choose a higher intensity exercise like a stairstepper, jogging/running, Nordic track, kick boxing, or a spin class.

Some people who are either short on time or who have difficulty exercising for a full 45 to 60 minutes ask me if it is possible to do more shorter sessions over the course of the day. There is mounting evidence that a few short exercise sessions during the day provide the same blood pressure–lowering and weight loss impact as does one long session. This knowledge allows a person to progress more quickly through the initial conditioning and improvement stages of developing an exercise program.

DEVELOPING YOUR EXERCISE PROGRAM

Now you that you are ready to begin an exercise program, it's important to plan it out. The American College of Sports Medicine (ACSM) defines three stages of an aerobic exercise program: an initial conditioning stage; an improvement stage; and a final or maintenance stage, which is meant to last a lifetime. The ACSM also provides guidelines regarding the expected rate of progression. Remember, these are only guidelines.

It is generally recommended that the initial conditioning stage should last four to six weeks; the improvement stage, between twelve and twenty-four weeks; and the maintenance phase, a lifetime. Many people continue to become more fit during the maintenance phase, and it is during this phase that new types of exercise may be attempted. People who enjoy a challenge may consider training for a road race or bike race. As you progress through the stages, remember that the recommended rate of progression is not absolute. Some people will get bored with the initial conditioning phase and will want to move on to the improvement phase within two weeks, while others might spend twelve to sixteen weeks working on the initial conditioning phase. Either approach is fine. You know your body best. I remind you that it is important to discuss any new exercise program and your plans for progression with your personal physician.

The next few pages will help you plan such an exercise program. The focus here will be on a walking program, but other forms of aerobic exercise are perfectly acceptable as long as they allow you to achieve your desired heart rate and fitness goals. Table 4.2 outlines the initial conditioning stage of your exercise plan. Your target heart rate is 50 to 60 percent of your MHR.

Table 4.2 Developing an Exercise Plan: The Initial Conditioning Stage

WEEKS	FREQUENCY	INTENSITY	TIME
1–2	3–5 times a week	50–60% MHR★	15 minutes
3–4	3–5 times a week	50–60% MHR	15–18 minutes
5–6	3–5 times a week	50–60% MHR	18–20 minutes

★MHR = maximum heart rate

During this initial conditioning phase two things are crucial: consistency and patience. You will not improve if you only exercise once a week. Conversely, if you jump into exercise and try to work out seven days a week, 60 minutes per session, you may well experience an overuse injury. I suggest the following program.

Try to push for five times a week if your goal is weight loss. If your only goal is blood pressure reduction, three times a week, up to 20 minutes per session, is sufficient at this stage. The information in Table 4.3 gives you your target heart rate range for the initial conditioning phase.

You are now ready to move to the improvement stage, which

Table 4.3 Target Heart Rates for the Initial Conditioning Phase

AGE	50–60% MHR	10-SECOND PULSE
20	100–120	17–20
25	98–117	17–20
30	95–114	16–19
35	92–111	16–19
40	90–108	15–18
45	88–105	15–18
50	85–102	14–17
55	82–99	14–17
60	80–96	13–16
65	78–93	13–16
70	75–90	12–15
75	72–87	12–15
80	70–84	11–14
85	68–81	11–14

on average will last between twelve and twenty-four weeks. During the improvement stage it is up to you to determine your goals. If weight loss is important to you, I suggest working up to a frequency of six to seven sessions per week. If blood pressure reduction is your only concern, you may continue to exercise only three times a week during this phase. Likewise, let your body guide you regarding intensity. It is perfectly acceptable to continue at 50 to 60 percent of the MHR during the improvement stage. Finally, almost everyone should aim to accumulate 30 minutes of exercise each day they exercise. This does not have to occur all at once; it might be accomplished as two 15-minute sessions or three 10-minute sessions. However, if weight loss is an objective, the goal should be to accumulate between 45 and 60 minutes nearly every day.

Tables 4.4 and 4.5 will help you to develop an exercise plan for the improvement stage.

Table 4.4 Developing an Exercise Plan: The Improvement Stage

WEEKS	FREQUENCY	INTENSITY	TIME
7–10	4–5 times a week	60–70% MHR	20 minutes
11–14	4–5 times a week	70–80% MHR	25 minutes
15–20	5–6 times a week	70–85% MHR	30 minutes
21–25	6–7 times a week	70–85% MHR	45–60 minutes

Table 4.5 Target Heart Rates for the Improvement Stage

AGE	60–85% MHR	10-SECOND PULSE
20	120–170	20–28
25	117–166	20–28
30	114–162	19–27
35	111–157	19–27
40	108–153	18–26
45	105–149	18–26
50	102–145	17–25
55	99–140	17–25
60	96–136	16–24
65	93–131	16–24
70	90–128	15–23
75	87–123	15–23
80	84–119	14–22
85	81–115	14–22

THE MAINTENANCE STAGE

The maintenance stage requires persistence and commitment. Now you have acquired the skills necessary to maintain an exercise program for life; staying committed is the challenge. Some people find that working with a partner sustains their enthusiasm; others reward themselves with a prize if they accumulate a certain number of miles per month. For them, charting mileage is fun. One of my patients set a year-long goal to walk one thousand miles. She figured out that traveling south, one thousand miles would get her to St. Augustine, Florida. She plotted her mileage weekly and at the end of the year, she and her husband flew to St. Augustine, where she had a great time telling the locals about her long walk.

Another way to stay excited about exercise is to train for a worthy cause. Walking in the American Heart Association Walk or another charitable event is a great way to make your fitness benefit others as well as yourself.

Finally, depending on where you live, you must plan how you will continue to maintain your exercise program during the winter months. Many people purchase a treadmill, and this is an excellent idea. However, be sure to purchase an electric one. Self-propelled treadmills are very difficult to work with, and as a result people give up. Others join a gym in the winter or walk at a local mall or high school.

In general, during the maintenance stage you should plan on walking six to seven times a week at 70 to 85 percent of your MHR. Each session should last about 60 minutes. Again, you can customize this according to your fitness goals.

WARM-UP AND COOL-DOWN

Because you will want to continue your exercise program for the rest of your life, it is crucial to take steps to avoid injury. A warm-up and cool-down are two very important components of your exercise program. For many people who want to jump right in to an exercise routine, this can seem tedious. I assure you, it is essential.

The warm-up consists of a 5- to 10-minute period of either stretching or a less-intense version of your chosen exercise. I generally recommend a slow walk. This slow walk allows your body to reach your target heart rate (whatever it may be) safely and comfortably.

The cool-down helps slow your heart down gradually. Over the course of a 5- to 10-minute slow walk you should be able to bring your heart rate fairly close to your pre-exercise heart rate. Slowing your heart rate gradually helps prevent blood from pooling in your legs, greatly reducing the risk of fainting and lightheadedness. Stretching is also a good idea during the cool-down phase of your program.

Remember, the warm-up and cool-down phases of your exercise session do not count toward the total time exercising. If you are aiming for a 60-minute program, the warm-up and cool-down can add between 10 and 20 minutes.

BE PATIENT

I have saved my most important advice for the end of the chapter. As you embark on an exercise program, it is important to be patient with yourself. You may not have enjoyed exercise in the past; but if you give yourself eight weeks (get into the improvement stage), you will find that your body can do more than you ever thought it could. You will become proud of what you have accomplished. You may hate to admit it, but you will begin to enjoy walking (or biking or swimming—whatever exercise you have chosen). Even if you don't quite get to the point of liking exercise, consider what one of my patients told me: "There is nothing like having exercised." After a year of regularly working out, he still didn't enjoy the program, but he knew he needed it and was committed to continuing. He told me he routinely exercised first thing in the morning so that he could "get it over with" and start his day with a satisfying feeling of "having already exercised."

I hope it will be more enjoyable to you than it is to this man, but no matter how you accomplish it, exercise is crucial to good blood pressure control. Why not head out today to buy a good pair of walking shoes, the only thing you need to get started on that trip toward better health?

Chapter 5

❧

Weight Loss

Losing weight, properly done, will not only lower blood pressure but can lower cholesterol, improve diabetes, decrease the risk of arthritis, and generally improve a person's sense of well-being. How do you determine if you need to lose weight? Actually, you just know. But since we all like to work from a rule, Table 5.1 (although not as precise as the Body Mass Index discussed earlier in this book) may be helpful.

For example, a woman who is five feet seven inches tall should ideally weigh 135 pounds and a man of the same height should weigh 147 pounds. You don't need to be slavish about it, however. Adjusting for your frame (small, medium, large) means you can weigh a bit less if you are small-boned and a bit more if you are large.

Table 5.1 Determining Ideal Weight

	MEN	**WOMEN**
First five feet of height	105 pounds	100 pounds
Every inch over five feet add	6 pounds	5 pounds

Once formal education is completed, the average American gains about a pound a year, and so this may be the best reason to go on for your doctorate (just kidding). As I mentioned earlier, Kannel and colleagues have found that each 10-pound weight gain translates into a 4.5 mmHg rise in systolic blood pressure. Thus, a person of fifty (thirty years beyond high school graduation) may have put on 30 pounds in those years with a corresponding increase in systolic blood pressure of as much as 13.5 mmHg.

Weight loss has a wonderful effect on blood pressure. A loss of as little as 10 pounds can lower systolic blood pressure by about 8 mmHg and diastolic by 6.5 mmHg. Some recent studies have documented even more dramatic effects. This degree of weight loss is often enough to prevent the need for blood pressure medications altogether or, if medications are necessary, very small doses are often sufficient.

In the United States overweight has become the norm. With 25 percent of children and 54 percent of adults falling into the overweight or obese categories, we are in trouble. Americans are the only people in the world who have reduced the fat in their diets and still gained weight. What we have forgotten about is calories. Just because a bagel is essentially fat free doesn't mean you should eat two. Bagels purchased at a deli or donut shop don't come with labels, and they often have 400 calories each (before the margarine or cream cheese).

I have already mentioned the issue of exercise. We have become an increasingly sedentary society, and since your weight is a function of calories eaten and calories expended, lack of exercise is responsible for a large number of excess pounds. The first thing I do when working on weight loss with my patients is to take a weight and diet history. Please answer these questions yourself.

- How much did you weigh when you graduated from high school (or some other important event such as your wedding day)?

- How much would you like to weigh?
- When was the last time you were satisfied with your weight?
- How many times have you lost and gained weight in the last two years?
- How motivated are you to make changes in your lifestyle to achieve your weight goal?

The answers to these questions are very helpful to me as a physician. Someone who was thin until high school graduation is different from someone who has been overweight since the age of two or three. It doesn't mean that the two people will necessarily lose weight at different rates. The difference, I find, is mainly in their self-image and confidence. My job is to let both people know—often in different ways—that anyone can be successful.

The answer to the second question, "How much would you like to weigh?" is also very helpful. I think it is important to be realistic. A man who is 50 pounds over his ideal body weight and says that he intends to lose 70 pounds doesn't really know what his ideal body weight is. Likewise, a woman who needs to lose 30 pounds but says that four or five would be fine is also a little vague on where she should be. I encourage people to set attainable goals. In the last example, an initial weight loss goal of 5 pounds is perfectly appropriate as long as she is aware that once that is attained, she will need to set a new target.

The third question is also very important: A person who has never been satisfied with her weight may always disappoint herself. At some point, one has to be realistic. Sometimes I need to explain to my patients that the most important goal of weight loss is to improve health, not to fit into a size four dress or shrink waist size by three to four inches. When high blood pressure is a concern, weight loss can eliminate the need for blood pressure medications for some people and reduce the dose of medications for others. A wonderful side benefit may be looking better in and out of one's clothing.

When I ask, "How many times have you lost and gained weight in the last two years?" the answer helps me determine the most important time for close follow-up. People who have lost and regained weight a number of times in just two years will almost certainly lose weight on our diet, too. They are veterans. But because regaining the weight is also part of their pattern, close follow-up is required to prevent relapse. These people need to be convinced of the importance of regular weight checks once a weight goal is achieved.

It is also crucial for them to know how important exercise is in preventing relapse. I tell such patients that anyone can lose weight with a diet, but few people maintain it without regular exercise. If a person tells me he has made no attempt to lose weight or that he hasn't been able to focus on a diet for a sustained period of time in the past two years, then he needs lots of encouragement early on. This is especially true during the first few weeks of the diet while his body is getting used to having fewer calories per day.

"How motivated are you to make changes in your lifestyle?" may be my most important question. If a person cannot articulate her degree of motivation or describe the likely personal health benefits of weight loss, she may not be ready to make the attempt. I can try to help, but true motivation must come from within. Only then will you be strong enough to withstand the temptations along the way.

In our clinic at the New England Heart Institute, we see people with multiple risk factors for developing heart disease. These include not only high blood pressure, but diabetes, high cholesterol, and smoking. Most of our patients are overweight and many have already had a heart attack or stroke. For this reason we take a very aggressive approach to diet and weight loss. The New England Heart Institute Diet restricts not only sodium, but calories and fat as well. We find most women lose weight and lower their blood pressure and cholesterol on 1,200 calories, 27 grams of fat, and no more than 2,400 milligrams of sodium. Men are typically allowed 1,500 calories, 35 grams of fat, and 2,400 milligrams of sodium.

Table 5.2 Numbers of Daily Servings

FOOD GROUPS	RECOMMENDED NUMBER OF SERVINGS PER DAY	
	1,200 CALORIES	1,500 CALORIES
Starch/bread/cereal/pasta	5	6
Meat/fish/poultry (1 ounce per serving)	5	5
Vegetables	3	3
Fruits	3	4
Fats	1	2
Dairy/milk	2	2 1/2

Table 5.2 details the numbers of servings that should represent daily intakes of both 1,200 and 1,500 calories. Exhibit 5.1 illustrates sample meal plans to give you a feel for serving size and good choices. Since you will want to vary your diet, I suggest you try a variety of different fruits and vegetables. Likewise, different bread, cereal, fish, poultry, and meat choices will help keep things interesting. In my previous book, *Heart Fitness for Life*, I provide meal plans and eighty chef-tested recipes.

Exhibit 5.1 Sample Meal Plans

DAY 1

Breakfast

> 1/2 cup oatmeal (1 starch)
> 1 small orange (1 fruit)
> 8 ounces skim milk (1 dairy)

Lunch

> 2 slices whole grain bread (2 starches)
> 2 ounces turkey (2 meat)
> lettuce and tomato (free food)

carrot sticks (1 vegetable)
1 1/2 teaspoons low-fat mayonnaise (1/2 fat)
18 grapes (1 fruit)

Snack

1 cup red and yellow pepper slices (1 vegetable)

Dinner

1 cup rice (2 starches)
3 ounces skinless chicken, baked (3 meat)
1/2 cup cooked broccoli (1 vegetable)
spring greens (free food)
1 1/2 teaspoon low-fat salad dressing (1/2 fat)
1 cup cantaloupe (1 fruit)

Snack

1/2 cup fat-free frozen yogurt (1 milk)

If you are following the 1,500 calorie meal plan add:
1/2 cup oatmeal (1 starch)
1 cup blueberries
1 tablespoon diet margarine
4 ounces skim milk

Day 2

Breakfast

3/4 cup whole-grain cold cereal (1 starch)
1/2 banana (1 fruit)
4 ounces skim milk (1/2 milk)

Lunch

1 whole-wheat pita pocket (2 starches)
2 ounces chicken (2 meat)
lettuce and tomato (free food)
1 apple (1 fruit)
1/2 tablespoon reduced-fat mayonnaise (1/2 fat)
seltzer water, any flavor (free food)

Snack

> 1 orange or kiwi (1 fruit)
> 8 ounces 100 calorie yogurt (1 milk)

Dinner

> 3 ounces shrimp cocktail (3 meat)
> cocktail sauce (free food)
> 1/2 cup asparagus (1 vegetable)
> 1/2 cup rice (1 starch)
> 1/2 tablespoon light margarine (1/2 fat)
> greens and tomato (free food)
> 1 tablespoon fat-free dressing (free food)

Snack

> 1 1/2 graham crackers (1 starch)
> 4 ounces skim milk (1/2 milk)

If you are following the 1,500 calorie meal plan add:
> 1 slice whole-grain toast (1 starch)
> 1/2 banana (1 fruit)
> 1 tablespoon light margarine (1 fat)
> 4 ounces skim milk (1/2 milk)

DAY 3

Breakfast

> 1 whole-wheat English muffin (2 starches)
> 1 orange (1 fruit)
> 1/2 cup 100 calorie yogurt (1/2 milk)
> 2 teaspoons all-fruit jam

Lunch

> 1 1/2 cups low-salt minestrone soup (2 vegetables and 1 starch)
> 6 salt-free Saltines (1 starch)
> 1 cup watermelon (1 fruit)
> 1 glass water (free food)

Snack

> 1 apple (1 fruit)
> 4 ounces skim milk (1/2 milk)

Dinner

> 1 small potato, baked (1 starch)
> 5 ounces fresh flounder (5 meat)
> 1 cup steamed zucchini (1 vegetable)
> tossed green salad (free food)
> 2 tablespoons fat-free dressing (free food)
> 1 tablespoon light margarine (1 fat)
> 1 tablespoon fat-free sour cream (free food)

Snack

> 1 cup fat-free frozen yogurt (1 milk)

If you are following the 1,500 calorie meal plan add:
> 1 cup whole-grain cereal (1 starch)
> 1 peach (1 fruit)
> 4 ounces skim milk (1/2 milk)
> 1 teaspoon olive oil (1 fat)

WEIGHT LOSS AIDS

Occasionally the question of a weight loss aid comes up in our clinic. There are a number of prescription medications currently available to promote weight loss. These include phentermine (Ionamin), sibutramine (Meridia), and orlistat (Xenical). In addition to the prescription medications, there are a number of so-called "fat burners" which are available without a prescription. Let's first review the medications that are available by prescription and then the over-the-counter therapies.

Prescribing a medication for weight loss should never be done lightly. The medication may or may not be effective in a given situation, and they all have potential side effects.

You may remember that dexfenfluramine (Redux) was taken off the market in 1997 when heart valve abnormalities were discovered in a number of people, some of whom were on the medication for as little as a few months. Not only was Redux a serotonin reuptake inhibitor, it was also a serotonin releasing agent. The end result was a dramatic rise in serotonin levels in brain synapses as well as in the bloodstream. In the brain, elevated serotonin levels suppress a person's appetite, which naturally results in weight loss. So far, so good. Unfortunately, many scientists believe the dramatic increase in blood seratonin is the cause of the heart valve abnormalities. In addition, the other potential and possibly deadly side effect of Redux was primary pulmonary hypertension (PPH), a restrictive lung disease. Symptoms of PPH can include shortness of breath, reduced ability to exercise, and edema (fluid buildup) in the legs. There is no doubt that Redux was an effective weight loss medication, but the side effects were unacceptable. Ultimately, Redux was removed from the market, but not until more than 18 million prescriptions for it had been written.

Ionamin, a sympathomimetic amine that behaves very similarly to amphetamines (speed), is a weight loss medication that is still available by prescription. Because Ionamin has the potential to significantly elevate blood pressure, I do not routinely recommend it. Other side effects of concern include palpitations, generalized anxiety, dry mouth, trouble sleeping, and constipation.

Meridia is a relatively new weight loss drug. Although it shares some properties with Redux, it leads to much lower brain and blood levels of serotonin and therefore appears to be much safer. Like Redux, Meridia is an appetite suppressant. Although I have prescribed this drug for a limited number of my patients, I would not recommend it to persons with high blood pressure. Meridia, like Ionamin, has the potential to raise blood pressure. In some patients it is only a matter of a few points, but in others it can be quite substantial. Where high blood pressure is already an issue, I don't think it wise to prescribe it.

Very recently the lipase inhibitor orlistat, marketed as Xenical, has come on the market. Xenical works by inhibiting the ability of lipases to function. Lipases are enzymes within the intestine that facilitate the breakdown and absorption of fat. Xenical inhibits the absorption of approximately 30 percent of the fat a person takes in. If fat is not absorbed, it must go somewhere. I am sure you can guess where that is. The major side effect of Xenical, then, is abdominal cramping and diarrhea. In the majority of patients, this side effect is most pronounced when they first begin the medication and learn how much fat they can safely have without spending the evening in the bathroom. Although all the studies with Xenical were done with participants taking the medication at a dose of 120 mg three times a day, we have had success with patients taking the medication only once a day.

We generally suggest this because our patients tend to eat a very low-fat breakfast and lunch. It makes little sense to take this drug, which works by preventing fat absorption, when no fat has been consumed. But even people on a low-fat diet generally eat some fat at the evening meal. In our practice, one pill at the evening meal generally results in a weight loss of about 10 pounds over the course of six months. This has been enough to lower the blood pressure in some of our patients to the point where blood pressure medications could be discontinued.

Our experience with Xenical is quite similar to what has been reported in the scientific literature. After one year on Xenical, people with elevated blood pressure (greater than 140/90) experienced a drop in systolic blood pressure of 11 mmHg and a fall in diastolic blood pressure of 8 mmHg. The drop in blood pressure is due solely to the weight loss effect of the drug. Xenical will not affect blood pressure unless a person loses weight.

Bill is one of our favorite patients. When we met him he was forty-seven and had already had a heart attack and an angioplasty. At that time he had high blood pressure, high cholesterol, and was obese. (At six feet tall he weighed 256 pounds.) Having been overweight his entire adult life, Bill knew his weight was his biggest problem. He freely admitted binge eating after his wife and children had gone to bed. He explained that while he had no difficulty sticking with a sensible low-fat, low-calorie diet the entire day, he lost all control after dinner. And late at night, it was not uncommon for him to eat a bowl of ice cream and twelve to fourteen Oreo cookies, washed down with two to three glasses of milk. Intellectually, Bill knew what to do, and his family was very supportive. Bill knew that if he didn't get things under control soon, he might not be so lucky with his next attack. He wanted to be around when his daughters graduated from high school and college and to see them married and settled. He wanted to be able to travel with his wife when he retired.

We worked with Bill for two years. He changed a few things in his diet, but lost only a total of three to four pounds. As for exercise, while he always left our office with good intentions, he never quite followed through with the walking program we outlined. We normalized his cholesterol, but it took two drugs, and his blood pressure still wasn't perfect despite three medications.

When Xenical came on the market, I felt it was worth a try. I told Bill it wasn't a magic bullet but that it might help. I also warned him that he was likely to experience abdominal cramping and diarrhea if he kept up his Oreo cookies and ice cream ritual. Bill decided to take the Xenical with his evening snack. He found it served two purposes: It acted as behavior modification in a capsule (he didn't want diarrhea), and it prevented the absorption of 30 percent of the fat he ate with his bedtime snack.

Bill took the scientific approach to the new drug. The first night he tested it by eating his usual snack and taking the medicine. The result was a night in the bathroom. After that he forced himself to take the Xenical prior to his snack and, the all-night experience quite vivid in his memory, he found he was able to limit himself to two to three Oreos. Oreos are still not a great choice, but I am the first to admit that three is better than fourteen.

He has now lost 10 pounds, gotten rid of one of his three blood pressure medications, and has been able to cut back on his cholesterol medication, too. He is still about 50 pounds above his ideal body weight, but if he can sustain this loss he is going to be at much lower risk of a heart attack or stroke. Interestingly, since Bill has lost weight he is much more willing to exercise. For the last three months he has walked thirty minutes per day at least six days a week. The exercise should allow him to maintain his weight loss and improved blood pressure and cholesterol levels.

Over-the-Counter Weight Loss Supplements

Millions of Americans try over-the-counter weight loss supplements. It is a billion-dollar industry, and there are literally dozens of weight loss supplements on the market. They go by names such as Fat Burner, Exercise in a Bottle, Pyruvate Punch, Ultra Burn, Ultra Lean, Super Fat Control, and Thin-Thin. Once again, it is crucial for you to know what you are putting into your body and whether or not it works.

Do they work? In general, they do not (except perhaps by the indirect route: i.e., spending your money on the drugs leaves you with less to waste on donuts and french fries). The exceptions to this rule are preparations containing ephedrine (ma huang), a Chinese herb. The problem with ma huang or ephedrine is that it has been linked to kidney failure, seizures, strokes, chest pain, and to about thirty-six documented deaths.

Most of the weight loss supplements boast of a "key ingredient" responsible for their fantastic weight loss properties. Some of these ingredients include pyruvate, conjugated linoleic acid (CLA), and hydroxycitric acid (HCA).

Pyruvate is, not surprisingly, found in Pyruvate Punch. It is also the key ingredient in Exercise in a Bottle. Manufacturers claim that clinical trials have proven pyruvate to be dramatically superior to placebo. In fact, clinical trials found that dieters who took 30 grams of pyruvate a day (costing about $300 per month) lost an average of 3 1/2 pounds more than dieters taking placebo. That's about $86 a pound.

Conjugated linoleic acid (CLA), a substance found in meat and milk, was first discovered by Dr. Michael Pariza of the University of Wisconsin. Because it appeared to increase muscle and decrease fat in animals, it was tested in four hundred obese people. Obese volunteers took either 3 grams of CLA a day or placebo. Unfortunately, after nine months those in the CLA group had lost no more weight than had those in the placebo group. Because of this finding the study was terminated.

Hydroxycitric acid (HCA) comes from a tropical fruit called *Garcinia cambogia*. Because citric acid has a role in converting the calories we eat to stored fat, scientists thought that HCA, which is a modified form of citric acid, might prevent this action. Unfortunately, in animal studies performed by Hoffmann-La Roche, HCA proved to be quite toxic. Most notable was a shrinking of testicular size. Because of this issue the drug company decided not to proceed with further testing of HCA.

Nonetheless, HCA is on the market and is found in such "fat burners" as Citrimax and Citrin. With the possible risks associated with HCA, one would hope that it would at least live up to weight loss claims. Unfortunately, the longest study (twelve weeks) of HCA found that the forty-two patients taking it lost only 2 pounds less than the forty-two people taking the placebo: Placebo takers lost 9 pounds, those taking HCA only lost 7.

Overall your best bet in terms of weight loss is to eat fewer calories and exercise more. By doing so you will feel better, your blood pressure is likely to fall, and you won't have to worry about potential long-term side effects.

Is dieting hard? Just last week one of my patients came for his appointment. I hadn't seen him in four months. He had lost 15 pounds, which he had been trying to do for the last three years. Somewhat amazed, I asked Ed what had happened. How had done it? He told me that at our previous visit I had finally gotten through to him. What did I say? I didn't remember anything special or different about our last visit. He told me I said, "Ed, this isn't going to be easy. The first few weeks of any lifestyle change are always the hardest. It is likely that you will be a little grumpy and hungry. You are going to have to live with it. But it will get easier."

Once he mentioned this I remembered the conversation. I actually thought he had been a little annoyed with me at our last visit and I told him so. I knew he hadn't liked what I had said, but he told me I was right on the money. He went on to tell me that he had gone home and discussed the visit with his wife, who said, "You know, Ed, Dr. McGowan is right—you need to be a little more patient and persistent with your approach to diet and exercise. You have to be in it for the long haul if you want the changes to stick."

Ed told me that once he developed a new mindset, he was off and running. Yes, he was a little grumpy for a couple of weeks, but that had passed. At our visit Ed had a lot to be proud of: His weight had fallen by 15 pounds; his systolic blood pressure was down to 128; his diastolic had gone from 88 mmHg to 78mmHg; and his triglycerides were down from 250 mg/dl to 135 mg/dl. Overall he felt stronger and more confident in his work. As a salesman, Ed is constantly meeting new clients. At his new weight he simply thinks he makes a better impression. I know I was impressed.

CHAPTER 6

es

YOU CAN QUIT SMOKING!

For a long time we didn't think cigarette smoking had much effect on blood pressure. We now know otherwise. Smoking a cigarette increases blood pressure for about fifteen to thirty minutes. This is a significant amount of time for one cigarette, but it took us quite a while to put two and two together. Most people don't smoke in the fifteen to thirty minutes before they get their blood pressure measured in the doctor's office. The last chance you get is probably in the car on the way to your appointment. Then it is time to find a parking spot and walk into the doctor's office. There you register and fill out insurance forms, after which you may sit in the waiting room for a minimum of fifteen minutes and often more in the exam room. By the time your blood pressure is being taken, the effect of the cigarette in the car is long gone. (Of course, if the wait was a long one, your blood pressure might be up for an entirely different reason!)

So it really wasn't until ambulatory blood pressure monitoring became possible that we were able to accurately assess the effect of smoking on blood pressure. With an ambulatory monitor, which is worn over the course of twenty-four hours, blood pressure is automatically taken and recorded throughout the day. The person wearing the monitor is instructed to keep a diary of activities including meals, exercise, emotional upsets, smoking, watching television, and so on. By correlating activities as noted in the diaries with the blood pressure readings throughout the day, researchers were finally able to see the impact of a single cigarette and the actual number of minutes blood pressure remained elevated after each one. For the average pack-a-day smoker, this is no small matter. A single cigarette is bad enough—a pack a day is responsible for up to ten hours of elevated blood pressure.

So how do you go about quitting? Let me say from the outset, quitting smoking is one of the hardest things you will ever do—but it is also one of the most rewarding. Without even meeting you, I can say you are probably fed up with the habit yourself. The fact is, at least 80 percent of adult smokers desperately want to quit. Intellectually, just knowing that your cigarette smoking may be the cause of your high blood pressure should be enough to motivate you to quit. Some people are able to quit when faced with the health consequences of the habit; but for most people, the information just makes them feel worse, not more resolved.

The truth is, you can become a nonsmoker. It won't be easy, but there are things you can do to make the road a little smoother. An important first step is to determine just how addicted you are. I generally ask my patients to take the assessment in Exhibit 6.1.

Question 3 of the Fagerstrom Nicotine Dependency Assessment may seem a little confusing. It is based on the fact that studies have shown smokers who need that first morning cigarette are the most highly addicted. Because the level of nicotine in your bloodstream declines dramatically as you sleep, highly addicted people "need" a cigarette the minute they wake in the morning. This sends the level of nicotine in the bloodstream up and allows the smoker to start the day. If this is your situation, you can still become a nonsmoker, but it will be more difficult for you than it will be for a person who can wait until noon before having a cigarette.

Exhibit 6.1 Fagerstrom Nicotine Dependency Assessment

1. How soon after you wake do you smoke your first cigarette?

0 points	1 point	2 points
After 1/2 hour	Within 1/2 hour	—

2. Do you find it difficult to refrain from smoking where it is forbidden, such as in the library, theater, doctor's office?

0 points	1 point	2 points
No	Yes	—

3. Which cigarettes would you hate to give up the most?

0 points	1 point	2 points
Any other than the first in the the morning	The first in the morning	—

4. How many cigarettes do you smoke a day?

0 points	1 point	2 points
1–15	16–25	26 or more

5. Do you smoke more in the morning than the rest of the day?

0 points	1 point	2 points
No	Yes	—

6. Do you smoke if you are so ill that you are in bed most of the day?

0 points	1 point	2 points
No	Yes	—

7. How often do you inhale the smoke from your cigarette?

0 points	1 point	2 points
Never	Often	Always

Reprinted from: Fagerstrom KO. Measuring degree of physical dependence on tobacco smoking with reference to individualization of treatment. *Addictive Behaviors.* 1978 (3): 225–241. With kind permission from Elsevier Science Ltd., The Boulevard, Langford, Kidlington OX51GB, UK.

Scoring the assessment is straightforward. Determine your total number of points from questions 1 through 7. A score of 6 or higher indicates strong nicotine dependency. In general, I suggest that people with such a score strongly consider using a smoking cessation aid. This may be the oral medication bupropion (also known as Zyban or Wellbutrin), nicotine gum, patch, nasal spray, or inhaler. A smoking cessation support group or structure class is also very helpful. If your score is 5 or less, you are not as highly addicted. Although a smoking cessation aid might be helpful, it may not be absolutely essential.

Now that you have assessed your level of addiction, it is also important to assess your motivation to quit. You can probably list a host of reasons in favor of quitting: Your blood pressure will go down. Your protective cholesterol (the HDL or high-density lipoprotein cholesterol) will go up. You will decrease your risk of heart disease, stroke, bladder cancer, and lung cancer. You are much less likely to develop chronic lung disease. You will improve your ability to exercise. Your self-esteem will rise. Your children and/or significant other will be proud of you. You won't have to spend another winter standing outside your office building with all the other banished smokers. You will get a break on life insurance. You will smell better. Food will taste better. Your ceilings will not need to be painted as frequently.

Whatever your motivating force, it is important that you be very committed, because there will be lots of tough moments, especially in the first month. This is the most difficult time, because you have not only the physical symptoms of withdrawal to contend with, but the psychological as well. After a month, all the unpleasant withdrawal symptoms (irritability, trouble sleeping, difficulty concentrating, cough, constipation, chest pain, and shakiness) are gone. "Only" the psychological addiction remains. This is what is responsible for still wanting a cigarette even years after quitting.

One of my patients tried at least a dozen times to quit smoking, and now he's been off cigarettes for four years. He told me that every time he gets the urge for a cigarette (for him it is always at a restaurant after a very satisfying meal), he tries to remember how tough that first month off cigarettes was for him and his family. Not wanting to relive that month is his motivation. I think he is only half-joking when he says his wife would divorce him if she had to go through another month like that.

Once you have determined that you are highly motivated, you are ready for the next step—setting a quit date. Ideally you should give yourself two weeks to prepare. The first week is spent looking at your current smoking habits. Although you might want to cut back during this week, I generally advise that you simply record each cigarette you smoke. Attach an index card to your package of cigarettes; each time you smoke, write down the time of day and what you were doing. It is also helpful to note how badly you wanted the cigarette. At the end of seven days look at your seven index cards. Do any patterns emerge? Do you smoke more when you are stressed? Bored? Tired? Hungry? After meals? With alcohol? With coffee or tea? What cigarettes do you want the most, and what cigarettes are purely out of habit? Pick out the five cigarettes you want most per day. For the next week, smoke only the five most important cigarettes of the day. You should also spend this week getting ready to become a nonsmoker by doing the following:

- Tell your friends and family when you will become a nonsmoker.
- Practice sitting in the nonsmoking section of a restaurant.
- Stock up on sugar-free hard candies and sugar-free freeze pops.
- Pick up a few jigsaw puzzles; buy yourself a new low-stress computer game; enroll in a night course requiring you to use

your hands (woodworking, painting, quilting); get out your old board games and find a nonsmoking partner.

- Stock up on herbal teas and bubble bath.
- Buy a few new relaxing CDs.
- Declare your home a smoke-free zone as of your quit date. Toss out your ashtrays.
- Clean out all the ashtrays in your car. Fill the ashtrays with cinnamon-flavored toothpicks.
- Have your car detailed so that it smells clean and fresh.
- Have your drapes and carpets cleaned.

Now you are ready! I recommend you quit smoking on a Saturday (or if you work on Saturdays, quit on a day off). Try to plan a very relaxed day for your first day as a nonsmoker. It will be helpful for you to plan a day of smoke-free activities: go to a movie, go to the library, go for a long walk. Tell your friends and family that you are quitting cigarettes and ask for their help and encouragement.

The first four weeks off cigarettes are the hardest. You are likely to be irritable and anxious, especially when you get the urge to smoke. Those first few weeks you will no doubt spend a great deal of time thinking about cigarettes—many people even dream about them. An intense craving for a cigarette is a signal to hold on tight and recognize what is happening—intense cravings only last a couple of minutes. During that time try:

- Going for a walk or bike ride.
- Brushing your teeth.
- Taking ten deep breaths in through your nose and letting them out slowly through your mouth.
- Sucking on sugar-free hard candy.
- Drinking a glass of water.
- Calling a friend.

Just a few more words on how you might feel during your first few weeks as a nonsmoker. Aside from feeling irritable, many of my patients complain that they feel washed out and extremely tired, but unable to sleep well. Many also mention that instead of getting rid of their smoker's cough, it has actually gotten worse. All of these symptoms are common and will get better.

Since nicotine is a stimulant, it makes sense that when your body is abruptly cut off you might feel very tired. But why should you have trouble sleeping? The answer to this is less clear, but it appears that nicotine has a strong influence over sleep patterns and that abrupt withdrawal can cause marked insomnia even in people who feel very tired and want to sleep. The insomnia tends to be short-lived, generally no longer than a week or so.

The reason the smoker's cough increases is that the cilia (small filamentous tubules that line healthy lung passages), which have been destroyed by years of smoking, quickly begin to grow back (more hopeful evidence of the body's ability to heal itself!); as they do, a cough can develop. In fact, this itself can help get rid of some of the residual debris in the lungs that has built up over years of smoking. The cough is typically very short-lived.

Many people also tell me that when they quit smoking they suddenly developed constipation. At first I didn't really pay much attention to this complaint, but after hearing it a few times I went to the medical literature and found that it is, in fact, true. Since this is the last thing you need to add to your list of problems as you quit smoking, be proactive. Increase exercise as you quit. Exercise is known to stimulate bowel activity. Increase your consumption of high-fiber foods such as fruits, vegetables, and oat bran. Drink lots of water. I recommend at least four pieces of fruit per day (good choices include oranges and apples), and try to include four servings of vegetables too (good choices are raw carrots, red or green pepper, and broccoli). Finally, set drinking eight glasses of water as your daily goal. If you are eating fruits and vegetables, drinking water, and exercising, you will also be less likely to gain weight.

For many people, the tips outlined above are helpful but not sufficient to achieve their goal of a smoke-free life. If you scored above six on the Fagerstrom Nicotine Dependency Assessment you may well benefit from a smoking cessation aid. In addition to nicotine replacement (gum, patch, inhaler, and nicotine nasal spray), smokers now have another option: bupropion (wellbutrin or Zyban). This choice may be even more beneficial than the nicotine replacement. Bupropion may be used alone or in combination with nicotine replacement. The nicotine patch, a popular form of nicotine replacement, is currently available without a prescription. There are several different brands including Habitrol (Ciba-Geigy), Nicoderm (Hoechst Marion Roussel, Inc.), Nicotrol (Pharmacia AB), and Prostep (American Cyanamid Co.). With the exception of Prostep, which comes in only two doses, each patch comes in three dosing levels. The idea is to gradually reduce your nicotine exposure over a period of eight to sixteen weeks.

Instructions on exactly how to use the patch are provided with each package. With the nicotine patch people break the smoking habit in two steps. First they get rid of the repetitive hand-to-mouth ritual, then they gradually reduce their dependence on nicotine by slowly withdrawing from it. Studies have shown that the "quit rate" is higher with the patch than quitting cold turkey. In addition, it appears that people who use the patch gain less weight as they quit.

The patch is generally placed on the upper, outer aspect of a person's arm (over the tricep muscle), on the upper aspect of the chest wall (above the breasts), or on the upper part of the back. Since some people are sensitive to the adhesive in the patch and can develop a skin rash, I recommend placing the patch on the left arm on even days of the month and on the right on odd days. Or you can consider rotating from the right arm to the chest wall to the left arm and then the back. If your skin is sensitive to the patch or if you want to try an alternate form of nicotine replacement, consider the use of nicotine gum, nicotine nasal spray, or the new Nicotrol inhaler. I find the gum and inhaler especially useful for people who really need to have something in their mouths.

The nicotine gum is available as 2 or 4 milligram doses. I think the 4 milligram dose provides better relief of withdrawal symptoms than does the 2 milligram dose. The gum comes with instructions, but a few points are still worth noting, since in my experience many people use this gum improperly. It works by allowing you to absorb nicotine through your gums, so it needs to be in contact with them. After chewing for about twenty seconds or so, park the gum between your cheek and gums where the nicotine will be easily absorbed and your craving diminished. Eating or drinking, especially carbonated beverages, while you are chewing the nicotine gum diminishes your ability to absorb the nicotine.

The nicotine spray has been proven to aid in smoking cessation. There have been three large trials comparing the nicotine spray (marketed by McNeil Consumer Products) with a placebo spray. Patients were followed for one year, and at each time point examined, the quit rate was twice as high for those using the nicotine spray.

The usual dose of the Nicotrol nasal spray is two sprays (one in each nostril). I ask my patients not to sniff, swallow, or inhale through the nose as they are spraying. I also ask them to tip their head back slightly as they deliver the spray. The two sprays provide 1 mg of nicotine. After two sprays, blood levels of nicotine rise rapidly. Maximum blood levels are achieved for most people between four and fifteen minutes after a dose. For many people, a 1 mg dose allows them to achieve the same nicotine blood level as after smoking a cigarette. People with a cold or runny nose will take about 30 percent longer to achieve a similar blood nicotine level because of the delay in absorption.

I generally ask my patients to start out with one to two doses per hour, which can be increased up to a maximum recommended daily dose of 40 mg (eighty sprays). I also recommend no more than five doses (ten sprays) over the course of an hour. After ten to twelve weeks of use, taper the use of the spray. Many people start by cutting their dose to one spray instead of two, then work on increasing the length of time between sprays.

Based on the results of a study published in the *British Journal of Medicine*, I now use the spray as a follow-up to the nicotine patch. In this study, entitled "Nicotine Nasal Spray with Nicotine Patch for Smoking Cessation: A Randomised Trial with Six-Year Follow-Up," Dr. T. Blondal and colleagues found that twice as many people were able to remain smoke free for six years when they were treated with a nicotine patch in decreasing dose for five months, followed by a year in which the nicotine spray was made available—versus five months of the patch, followed by the availability of a placebo spray. I tell my patients that they can continue to use the nicotine spray for as long as they need it. It has been my experience that many patients will use it once or twice a week for as long as a year or two, and that many keep it with them for even longer "just in case." I recommend using the nicotine spray following the nicotine patch, along with the gum, a nicotine inhaler (see below), or bupropion (see below). I would not recommend it be used at the same time as the patch, since the patch is worn continuously.

In terms of side effects from the Nicotrol nasal spray, almost everyone complains of nasal irritation. This improves over time, but can be troublesome. Other complaints include runny nose, throat irritation, watering eyes, sneezing, and cough.

The new nicotine inhaler holds promise for people who not only are addicted to cigarettes, but also need the repetitive hand-to-mouth ritual. Also marketed by McNeil Consumer Products Co., the Nicotrol Inhaler is available by prescription from your doctor. It consists of a mouthpiece and a plastic cartridge (which is attached to the mouthpiece) capable of delivering 4 milligrams of nicotine.

Ten puffs of the inhaler is roughly the equivalent of one puff on a conventional cigarette. Each cartridge is designed to be used for about twenty minutes of continuous puffing. You may use as many as twenty cartridges per day for about twelve weeks. After this, you should gradually reduce the number of cartridges per day. The Nicotrol Inhaler should be used for no longer than six months. Although the Nicotrol Inhaler is typically well tolerated, some people note slight irritation in the mouth and throat.

Many patients are surprised when I suggest that they use nicotine replacement for up to a year. They often comment that this seems like an awfully long time. It is important to remember that nicotine is a powerfully addictive drug. Although the physical addiction is over within a month, the emotional addiction can last for years. Having a "quick fix" nicotine replacement (such as the nicotine nasal spray) readily available may prevent relapse. This doesn't mean a person will use the "quick fix" frequently, but having it available can help prevent him from crumbling in a moment of weakness.

Recently bupropion (also known as wellbutrin or Zyban) has been found to be a very effective smoking-cessation tool. Bupropion was originally used as an antidepressant. Interest in this medication increased dramatically when it was also found to be useful in helping smokers kick the habit. One small study randomly assigned forty-two patients to receive either bupropion or placebo. At the end of two years 50 percent of those who were assigned to bupropion remained smoke-free, whereas all of those taking the placebo had resumed smoking.

Since bupropion is a prescription medication, you will be able to decide along with your physician if it is the right choice for you. People with a history of seizures should not take this medication. If you are already on another antidepressant, your doctor may choose to substitute bupropion for your current antidepressant. This, of course, may not always be appropriate.

When we prescribe bupropion we tell our patients to begin with 150 milligrams (one pill) once daily in the morning for three days. If you tolerate one pill per day, increase to 150 milligrams twice a day (two pills). Separate the pills by at least eight hours.

You should continue to smoke for the first week you are taking bupropion. On day eight, stop smoking. We recommend using bupropion for at least seven to twelve weeks. It is possible you may require this drug for longer than twelve weeks.

Side Effects: The most common side effects include dry mouth, constipation, headache, and trouble sleeping.

Precautions: As mentioned earlier, you should not take bupropion if you have a history of seizures. If you have been taking a monoamine oxidase inhibitor, you must discontinue this medication for at least two weeks prior to beginning bupropion.

The issue of continuing to smoke for the first week on bupropion is an important one. Before you can expect it to help you quit smoking, a certain level of this medication must build up in your bloodstream, and this occurs in about one week.

How effective are these medications? In a recent study published in the *New England Journal of Medicine*, Jorenby and collegues examined the impact of bupropion alone, the nicotine patch alone, or the two in combination as compared to placebo (sugar pill plus an inactive patch) in 893 smokers. All participants received counseling and supportive phone calls throughout the twelve-month study. At the end of the study the quit rate was 5.6 percent in the placebo group, 9.8 percent in the nicotine patch group, 18.4 percent in the bupropion alone group, and 22.5 percent in the combined treatment group. People treated with any form of nicotine replacement (that is, either the patch or bupropion) experienced less weight gain and fewer withdrawal symptoms.

No matter how you do it, quitting smoking is difficult, but you are worth the effort. Believe in yourself and just keep trying. If you slip up, rather than chastising yourself and wallowing in guilt (and more cigarettes), learn from the experience. Why did it happen? Try to make certain that you don't put yourself in that particular situation again.

However, suppose the situation that got you smoking again was a stressful interaction with your boss (or some other situation that you will not be able to just avoid as you become a nonsmoker). Here is a bit of advice my mother gave me when I had a difficult boss. As your boss is carrying on, try to picture him as a tiny baby with a messy diaper. I don't know why, but it helps. I think it helped me because it made me realize that we all start out the same way, and that just being a boss does not make one person superior to another. It also is just a funny thing to think about and can help you keep things in perspective: Do you really want to go back to smoking because of a stressful encounter with your boss?

As you become a nonsmoker you are likely to experience some setbacks along the way. Ultimately, if you continue to try, you will be successful. As a nonsmoker you will be much healthier. Not only will your blood pressure throughout the day improve, but your risk of lung disease, heart disease, and stroke—not to mention your risk of many forms of cancer—will decrease dramatically. You know you want to do it. I know you can.

CHAPTER 7

෨

AN OVERVIEW OF BLOOD PRESSURE MEDICATIONS

We have come a long way since the late 1940s when people with severe high blood pressure routinely died for lack of effective treatment. Before effective therapies became available, patients were treated with sedative medications, severe salt restriction, and even surgery to remove their adrenal glands. Finally in the 1950s, things started to change. We no longer use those early medications because they were fraught with severe side effects. They did, however, save lives and gave us the first hope that effective but less toxic medications would be discovered.

The only early blood pressure medications still in routine use are the diuretics (water pill), which were introduced in the late 1950s. In the mid '60s, beta-blockers were introduced to treat cardiac chest pain but were soon found to lower blood pressure as well. For many years, beta-blockers and diuretics were the mainstays of therapy. The early 1980s brought a virtual explosion of potent and well-tolerated blood pressure medications.

We now have nine classes of these medications:

1. Diuretics
2. Beta-blockers
3. Calcium channel blockers
4. Angiotensin-converting enzyme (ACE) inhibitors
5. Angiotensin-receptor antagonists
6. Alpha-adrenergic blockers
7. Alpha-beta receptor antagonists
8. Central and peripheral sympatholytics
9. Direct vasodilators

Each class lowers blood pressure by a different method. This is very important because many people who fail to respond to one class of drugs do beautifully with another.

Are some blood pressure medications inherently more effective than others? The answer is yes and no. In order to be approved by the Food and Drug Administration, a blood pressure medication must have been shown to lower blood pressure by at least 10 percent in the majority of people tested in clinical trials. Generally these trials include a cross section of the population (men, women, young, old, and people of different ethnic origins); however, in a particular individual, one class of blood pressure medication might lead to dramatically improved blood pressure readings, while another might have almost no impact.

CHOOSING THE CORRECT MEDICATION

How your physician decides which blood pressure medication will be best for you is an interesting mix of both general rules of thumb—and trial and error. Often a certain medication is chosen because it's been effective in a particular group to which you belong. For example, diuretic medications tend to be most effective in the elderly and in African Americans, while angiotensin-converting enzyme inhibitors (ACE inhibitors) are most useful in younger patients.

Another reason to choose one class of blood pressure–lowering medications over another is the side benefits of certain medications. Beta-blockers, for instance, can protect against chest pain in people with heart disease. Because they have also been shown to prolong life following a heart attack, they are the logical blood pressure–lowering choice in people with heart disease.

The same principle applies when considering which blood pressure medication to use in people with diabetes and/or a history of heart failure. In this situation, the logical choice is an ACE inhibitor, because this class of drugs has been shown to protect the kidneys of diabetic patients and reduce mortality in people with heart failure.

Even though your doctor can apply these and other guidelines as he makes an educated guess as to which blood pressure medication will be best for you, the first medication chosen may not do the trick. In general, I tell patients that it may take up to a year to achieve perfect blood pressure control. As drugs are being switched or dosages altered, your doctor may depend on you to monitor your own response with a home blood pressure monitor, thus saving you trips to the office for blood pressure checks.

CHOOSING THE CORRECT DOSE

Interestingly, when it comes to blood pressure–lowering medications many people are overdosed. In many situations the dose that is initially suggested by the manufacturer is found to be too high. The reason lies in the fact that drug companies understandably want their drug to be seen as working quickly in the vast majority of people. Typically, the initial recommended starting dose is that dose which was found to work successfully in the majority of a target population. Since there is truly a wide variation in response to different medications, placing everyone on the so-called "starting dose" of a medication will mean that many individuals will receive more drugs than needed. And these people may be the very ones who experience troublesome side effects.

For example, when hydrochlorothiazide (a diuretic) first came out, the starting dose was 200 mg per day. At such a high dose, one of the most alarming side effects is a dramatic reduction in the blood potassium level, which has the potential to cause deadly electrical disturbances in the heart. This side effect now almost never occurs because we generally treat people with just 12.5 mg per day.

The easiest solution to the problem of overdosing is to start at a level far below the standard starting dose of a medication and gradually increase it until the starting dose is reached. The gradual increasing of the medication can be done at home as long as the patient has an accurate home blood pressure cuff. Although this approach does not provide the immediate gratification of a prompt and dramatic reduction in blood pressure, it is, in the long run, probably the best approach because it allows the lowest effective dose of a medication to be used.

In addition to allowing individuals to be managed with low doses of medicine, this gradual upward titration of medications provides many patients with a correspondingly gradual reduction in blood pressure. This is particularly important for some individuals in whom a sudden drop of blood pressure may result in symptoms of weakness, fatigue, and dizziness. In part this is because one's body adjusts over time to high blood pressure and a sudden large drop results in a reduction in blood flow to the brain. A more gradual approach allows readjustment to a lower blood pressure without compromising this blood flow. (The human body, it must be noted, can "adjust" to many things. This does not imply, however, that those things are good for you!)

GETTING TO YOUR BLOOD PRESSURE GOAL

If you move gradually up to the starting dose of a medication, your doctor may be faced with the following situation: Your blood pressure has fallen with a particular drug but you have not yet achieved your blood pressure goal. At this point you and your doctor need to decide what to do. Should you further increase the dose of the drug? The upside of this approach is that you are still on only one blood pressure medication; the downside is that higher doses may mean more side effects.

Another approach would be to add a second medication. The advantage is that certain medicines work well together, and the starting doses of two medicines may actually be better in terms of side effects than a high dose of a single drug. The disadvantage of being on two blood pressure medicines is that it's sure to be more expensive than being on a single agent.

In addition, studies have shown that when people are asked to take two medications, they are less likely to do it. This is certainly understandable. It's harder to remember two pills instead of one, especially if they are taken at different times of the day. If your blood pressure improves but is not controlled on a low dose of one medication, you need to work with your doctor to determine which approach is going to be best for you. After all, you know yourself better than your doctor does. Although you can't predict if you will have a side effect from a certain medication, you do know if you would prefer to try one drug as opposed to two.

Remember, nothing is set in stone; and since it is likely that you will need blood pressure medications for the rest of your life, you might as well find the drug that best lowers your blood pressure and causes the least number of side effects. You should speak frankly to your doctor about this. Don't ever feel "locked in" to a certain medication. Don't settle for adequate control with some side effects until you have tried everything. After all, it is your body. You want to have optimum blood pressure, while feeling otherwise as good as you possibly can. Having said all this, it is true that there are some people in whom it is nearly impossible to fully normalize blood pressure, as well as some people who will have to put up with side effects. This should not, however, be the norm.

Another issue that needs to be considered as a blood pressure medication is chosen is how long it will exert its effect. The ideal drug is one that lowers blood pressure effectively for twenty-four hours. (Again, once-a-day medications are much easier to remember than those taken twice or three times a day.) Some drugs like amlodipine (Norvasc), a calcium channel blocker, and trandolapril (Mavik), an ACE inhibitor, actually lower blood pressure for longer than twenty-four hours. This may make these drugs a good choice for the 30 percent of people who miss at least one dose of their medication a week. Good twenty-four-hour coverage is essential given the fact that blood pressure routinely rises early in the morning. This early morning increase has been closely correlated with an increased risk of heart attacks in the early morning hours.

DIURETICS

Diuretics were first introduced in the late 1950s. They are frequently referred to as "water pills" because they promote increased urination. Diuretics truly revolutionized the care of people with high blood pressure and continue to be widely used today. The Systolic Hypertension in the Elderly Program (SHEP) found that in both men and women, the use of diuretics reduced the risk of heart disease by 25 percent and the risk of stroke by 36 percent.

Side Effects

As the SHEP trial was being analyzed, researchers questioned whether the degree of blood pressure reduction could predict the reduction in heart disease and stroke. Scientists found a very good correlation between a reduction in blood pressure and a reduction in stroke. Conversely, based on the degree of blood pressure reduction, a more substantial reduction in heart disease than was observed in the SHEP trial would have been expected. It is speculated that this disparity stems from some of the adverse effects of diuretics.

For example, some diuretics are known to cause a reduction in blood potassium levels, which can put a person at risk for the development of potentially deadly electrical disturbances in the heart's conducting system. Diuretics are also known to increase blood sugar levels. In some people, the increase in blood sugar can tip them over into diabetes. As you most likely know, people with diabetes are at high risk for developing heart disease. Diuretics can cause both triglycerides and LDL (or bad) cholesterol to rise. Elevated cholesterol levels also increase the risk of heart disease. The good news is that most of the adverse effects of diuretics are markedly reduced when the lowest possible dose is used. And the diuretic Lozol (indapamide) does not seem to cause the elevation in cholesterol or blood sugar seen with other diuretics. Finally, very recent evidence suggests that despite the fact that diuretics can cause an increase in blood sugar, they infrequently cause diabetes.

How Diuretics Work, and Who Should Take Them

As a rule, diuretics work by preventing the kidney from absorbing salt. The result is that a person taking a diuretic will lose salt and water from the kidney. This salt and fluid loss leads to a reduction in blood volume and hence reductions in blood pressure. One of the body's responses to the reduction in blood volume is to produce substances that result in a constriction or clamping down of blood vessels. Your body does this because it doesn't know whether you are losing blood volume because you have a massive cut and are bleeding or because you are taking a diuretic to lower your blood pressure. All your body knows is that something is changing and you are losing fluids. In reaction, it produces angiotensin II, a substance that makes the arteries constrict and tends to increase your blood pressure. People who produce lots of angiotensin II don't do very well on diuretics because, as you can imagine, this constriction of blood vessels actually leads to a rise in blood pressure. People who produce only small amounts of angiotensin II are likely to respond well to diuretics. This generally includes both elderly people and African Americans. Moreover, when compared to men, women do fairly well on diuretics because they have a reduced capacity to produce angiotensin II.

Types of Diuretics

Within the broad category of diuretics, there are three distinct groups depending on where in the kidney they exert their effect. These groups include:

1. Thiazides and thiazide-related compounds
2. Loop diuretics
3. Potassium-sparing diuretics

As mentioned below, the side effect profile of the diuretics differs among the groups. Table 7.1 lists current diuretics, their usual daily doses, and the number of doses required per day. As you will notice, sometimes two diuretics are combined for additive effects. Such combination preparations are also listed, and all of these contain at least 25 mg of hydrochlorothiazide. In my opinion, except for people who have very difficult-to-treat high blood pressure, doses greater than 12.5 mg are rarely necessary.

With such an array of drugs to choose from, it is fair to question just how your physician makes the decision to go with diuretics in the first place, and in the second, how she chooses one over another in your particular situation. As mentioned earlier, African Americans, women, and the elderly all tend to do well on diuretics.

Table 7.1 Diuretics and Dosages

DIURETIC	USUAL DAILY DOSE (MG) (NUMBER OF DOSES PER DAY)
Thiazides	
Bendroflumethiazide (Naturetin)	2.5–5.0 (1)
Benzthiazide (ExNa)	12.5–50 (1)
Chlorothiazide (Diuril)	125–500 (1)
Cyclothiazide (Anhydron)	0.5–2.0 (1)
Hydrochlorothiazide (Esidrix, HydroDiuril, Oretic, Microzide)	12.5–50 (1)
Hydroflumethiazide (Saluron, Diucardin)	12.5–50 (1)
Methyclothiazide (Enduron, Aquatensen)	2.5–5.0 (1)
Polythiazide (Renese)	1.0–4.0 (1)
Trichlormethiazide (Metahydrin, Naqua)	1.0–4.0 (1)
Thiazide-Related Compounds	
Chlorthalidone (Hygroton, Thalitone)	12.5–50 (1)
Indapamide (Lozol)	1.25–2.5(1)
Metolazone	
(Mykrox)	0.5–1.0 (1)
(Zaroxolyn)	2.5–10 (1)
Quinethazone (Hydromox)	25–100 (1)
Loop Diuretics	
Bumetanide (Bumex)	0.5–5.0 (2)
Ethacrynic acid (Edecrin)	25–100 (1)
Furosemide (Lasix)	20–480 (2)
Torsemide (Demadex)	5–40 (1)

Continued on page 106

Table 7.1 continued

Potassium-Sparing Diuretics	
Amiloride (Midamor)	5–10 (2)
Spironolactone (Aldactone)	25–100 (1–2)
Triamterene (Dyrenium)	50–150 (1–2)

Combination Preparations: *Dosing for combination preparations is listed as mg amount of the first drug in the combination followed by mg amount of the second drug.*

Amiloride HCL with hydrochlorothiazide (Moduretic)	5/50 (1)
Hydrochlorothiazide with triamterene	
(Maxzide-25 and Dyazide)	25/37.5 (1)
(Maxzide)	50/75 (1)
Spironolactone with hydrochlorothiazide (Aldactazide)	25/25–50/50 (1)

This is based on the fact that these groups of people tend to produce smaller amounts of angiotensin II than do middle-aged white males. So for biological reasons, diuretics are a good choice for these groups of patients.

Diuretics and Bone Health

One of the side effects of diuretics is a reduction in calcium loss from the kidney. Several studies have found that long-term exposure to diuretics can cause an increase in bone density and an overall reduction in hip fractures. I keep this in mind as I choose the best blood pressure medication for older women with osteoporosis (thin bones). Since a hip fracture can often spell the end of living independently for older women, this beneficial side effect can be of great importance.

Cost

Diuretics also tend to be very inexpensive, which is especially important for people on a fixed income who do not have insurance coverage of their medications. Although I hate to base any medical decision on money alone, this issue must be seriously considered. It might be that another blood pressure medication would actually suit a patient better than a diuretic, but if it is too expensive for him to buy it, it doesn't really matter how good it is.

Diuretics and Other Medications

If your doctor plans to put you on a diuretic, it is important for you to ask her if any of the other medications you currently take might decrease the ability of the diuretic to lower your blood pressure. Two common classes of medications used by people with arthritis or rheumatological problems do in fact decrease the overall effectiveness of diuretics. These include nonsteroidal anti-inflammatory medications such as Motrin or Naprosyn and steroids. This doesn't mean that your doctor should avoid trying a diuretic if you are on one of these medications; it just means that it might not work as well.

Diuretics and Potassium

Some of the negative side effects of diuretics can be avoided either by taking low doses or by moving from one class of diuretics to another. Almost anyone treated with thiazides, thiazide-related diuretics, or loop diuretics will experience a small drop in blood potassium level. In general, the higher the dose of the diuretic, the greater the risk. People on a high-salt diet are at higher risk of significant potassium losses. In general, the potassium loss is minor and not of clinical significance.

However, significant potassium depletion can lead to life-threatening electrical disturbances in the heart. Therefore, anyone started on one of the diuretic groups noted above should have a baseline potassium level drawn before beginning the medication and then a repeat level a week or so later. If potassium depletion does occur, the diuretic dose can be reduced. This may solve the problem and still provide good blood pressure reduction. Alternatively, a potassium supplement can be added or a switch to a potassium-sparing diuretic such as Midamor, Aldactone, or Dyrenium can be made. The potassium-sparing diuretics do not cause potassium loss; in fact, they may increase blood potassium levels.

Diuretics and Risk of Gout

All thiazides, thazide-related diuretics, and loop diuretics can increase uric acid levels in the blood. Marked elevations of uric acid are known to precipitate gout (painful, red, swollen joints—especially of the great toe—as a result of uric acid crystals exiting the blood and entering the joint space). Although I do not usually put people with a history of gout on thiazide diuretics, sometimes they are the only drugs that work.

William is one of my favorite patients. When I met him five years ago, he had already been in a wheelchair for twenty-five years following a college auto accident. He was sent to me because his primary care doctor was worried about his high blood pressure, high triglycerides (one of the blood fats that when elevated increases the risk of heart disease and stroke), and low HDL-cholesterol (the good cholesterol). Since his blood pressure was quite high (180/110 mmHg), I knew he needed a blood pressure medication right away.

Although we also set to work on diet, exercise, and alcohol restriction, I knew we simply didn't have the luxury of using only lifestyle measures for three to six months before adding a blood pressure medication. I knew (or thought I knew) I didn't want to use a diuretic. First of all, diuretics can raise triglycerides, which was one of the problems he already had. Second, William told me he had a history of gout (in his elbow and hands, and probably also in his toes, but he couldn't feel those).

Over the course of the next six months we tried many different medications (calcium channel blockers, ACE inhibitors, beta-blockers, angiotensin II receptor blockers, alpha 1 receptor blockers, and direct-acting vasodilators (all of which you will read about later in this chapter). Either they caused severe side effects or they simply didn't work. I was beginning to feel like a complete failure.

Finally I asked him if he would be willing to try a diuretic. I explained that he might develop gout and his triglycerides would likely increase. Actually, over the course of the previous six months as we had been trying various blood pressure medications, his triglycerides had fallen from 800 mg/dl down to 200 mg/dl (our goal was less than 150 mg/dl). This dramatic improvement was because he had lost 5 pounds, reduced his alcohol consumption to four drinks a week (down from ten), and started an upper body exercise program. Despite the improvement in his triglyceride level, his HDL-cholesterol remained very low. I knew we would have to tackle this as soon as his blood pressure was sorted out. William agreed to give HydroDiuril a try. Although I offered to start him on a medication called allopurinol to prevent the development of gout, he decided that he would chance it and only begin allopurinol if he developed gout. Well, believe it or not, two weeks later William's blood pressure was 130/80 mmHg on only 12.5 mg of HydroDiuril. He had no evidence of gout, even though his uric acid level had risen to 9.5 mg/dl (normal in our lab ranges from 3.1 to 8.0 mg/dl). His triglycerides, however, had increased slightly (to 250 mg/dl) and his HDL-cholesterol was still very low at 28 mg/dl (desirable is above 45 mg/dl). As I tried to decide how to manage his low HDL-cholesterol and high triglycerides, I weighed the risks of therapy against the possible side effects of the treatment. Overall, I knew William was at high risk of heart disease. He had a low HDL-cholesterol, high triglycerides, a bad family history (his father had died of a heart attack at the age of forty-two, and he himself was now forty-five years old), and he had only just gotten his blood pressure under control. Luckily he did not smoke or have diabetes.

I asked William if he thought there was any more he could do in terms of diet and exercise. He had made a great many dietary changes, and he was exercising one hour a day (upper body aerobic activity). He replied quite honestly that he was as good as he was going to get. I knew I would need to use a medication to lower his triglycerides and, more importantly, to raise his HDL-cholesterol level. My choices were Lopid, Tricor, or Niaspan. Tricor and Lopid, which are in the same family of medications, can dramatically lower triglycerides, but their impact on HDL is often less impressive. Nonetheless, because Niaspan can cause an increase in uric acid and precipitate gout as it lowers triglycerides and raises HDL, I thought it best to try one of these agents first. Unfortunately, while both agents lowered William's triglycerides dramatically, neither resulted in an improved HDL level.

Finally we steeled ourselves and began Niaspan. Niaspan is a long-acting preparation of the vitamin niacin. Taken once a day, it can often result in a dramatic improvement in HDL and triglycerides. Because it can also increase blood sugar and blood uric acid levels in much the same way as diuretics, I once again offered William the prophylactic allopurinol. Once again, he decided to take his chances.

The Niaspan had a profound impact: His triglycerides came down to 80 mg/dl while his HDL rose dramatically to 40 mg/dl. Luckily his blood sugar remained unchanged. Although his uric acid rose to 11.6 mg/dl, he still had no symptoms of gout.

Unfortunately, about ten weeks later William called me with the news I had been dreading. His elbow and hands were swollen, red, and painful. He had gout. He wondered if he could start the allopurinol. I explained that we would need to treat this attack of gout with anti-inflammatory medications. Once the attack was completely over, he could begin the allopurinol. Although I asked him to stop the Niaspan until the attack was over, he remained on the HydroDiuril.

Even though this set him back a month or so, we eventually got him on allopurinol. Once his uric acid was under control, we restarted the Niaspan, and his blood pressure, triglycerides, and HDL have been fine for the last four years with not a single episode of gout.

In William's case, in spite of being forced to use medications with all the wrong side effects, everything worked out in the end. I included this story because many people have a mental block where diuretics are concerned. The fact is, in many cases they work when other choices fail. This case also points out the importance of being patient. I tell people that although I am confident that their blood pressure will normalize, sometimes it may take as much as a year to accomplish.

You have probably noticed that I have not said much about the loop diuretics. In general these are used not so much for the treatment of high blood pressure but rather to promote fluid loss in people suffering from congestive heart failure. The loop diuretics tend to have a short duration of action, on the order of several hours, so they are not well suited to provide even blood pressure control over an entire day. When used twice a day, drugs like Lasix do, however, provide some blood pressure reduction. Of the loop diuretics, Demadex has the longest effect. In a patient who is also taking lithium, I would use a loop diuretic because the thiazide variety tends to cause a increase in lithium level that is highly undesirable. Potassium-sparing diuretics are currently needed only rarely. In the past, before we realized that in most people blood pressure could be handled with the use of very low doses of thiazides or thiazide-related diuretics, potassium wasting (meaning loss of potassium in the urine) was a big problem. Diuretics were created as the "potassium-sparing" solution (meaning preventing the loss of potassium in the urine). Nowadays, by using low doses of the thiazide diuretics, the potassium problem is pretty much avoided.

Nonetheless, in some situations potassium-sparing diuretics are still a good option. The most important thing to remember is that great care must be exercised if a potassium-sparing diuretic is used in conjunction with ACE inhibitors (ACE inhibitors are discussed later in this chapter). Both of these classes of blood pressure medications can cause potassium levels to increase, and the risk then becomes one of elevated rather than depressed potassium levels. Potassium is one of those things that must be in balance: Both too little or too much can result in rhythm disturbances in the heart.

Finally, my favorite diuretic is Lozol or indapamide. This thiazide-related diuretic does not have an adverse impact on either cholesterol levels or blood sugar.

BETA-BLOCKERS

Beta-blockers were first introduced in the early 1960s. Originally they were used to treat cardiac chest pain, but soon it became obvious that they also lowered blood pressure quite dramatically. During the '70s and '80s, beta-blockers and diuretics were the most commonly used blood pressure–lowering medications in the United States. One of the most important cardiac studies reported to date is the BHAT (Beta-blocker Heart Attack Trial). This trial tried to ascertain whether the use of propranolol (Inderol), a beta-blocker, prevented repeat heart attacks and death in people who had already suffered a heart attack.

Beta-Blockers Reduce the Risk of Heart Attacks

The study included almost four thousand people. It concluded that the use of propranolol (Inderol) reduced the risk of a recurrent heart attack by 23 percent and the risk of death by 26 percent. In a recent review of the literature, Soriano and colleagues found that the beta-blocker metoprolol (Lopressor, Toprol XL) provided the greatest protection against a recurrent heart attack. Based on this data, it is recommended that anyone who has had a heart attack be treated with a beta-blocker (regardless of blood pressure). As a result, if a person has both a history of heart disease *and* high blood pressure, the only logical choice is to use a beta-blocker.

How They Work

Beta-blockers work by blocking the beta receptors that are found on many of the body's organs. Beta receptors on the heart, lungs, and blood vessels allow them to receive messages from substances in the blood called catecholamines. Catecholamines are produced by the adrenal glands to help the body respond to both emotional and physical stress. For example, we have all heard stories of a man or woman being able to lift a car to save the life of a child pinned beneath it. The surge of superhuman strength comes from a surge in catecholamines (adrenaline). In a person with a normal heart this surge is helpful and allows him to do something he normally would never be able to do. In a person with a diseased heart the surge might cause a heart attack. This last example was an extreme one. Sometimes catecholamines are either slightly overproduced or exert an excessive impact. In such a situation, because of the impact catecholamines can have on the heart (see below), high blood pressure may result.

Catecholamines communicate with the heart via the beta-1 receptors and the heart responds by speeding up. Beta-blockers prevent the catecholamines from attaching to the beta-1 receptors. The result is a reduction in the heart rate as well as in the amount of blood pumped out of the heart with each beat, hence a corresponding reduction in blood pressure.

One of the ways the body responds to the drop in heart rate caused by the beta-blockers is to constrict the blood vessels of the hands and feet: These extremities then tend to feel excessively cold. This side effect of beta–blockers is a bigger problem for people living in cold climates and for those who have an underlying condition called Raynaud's disease. Since people with Raynaud's disease already have constriction of the blood vessels of the hands and feet, adding a beta–blocker may be disastrous, in rare cases leading to gangrene of a finger or toe.

The same catecholamines that bind to the beta–1 receptors of the heart also bind to the beta–2 receptors in the lung. Here the role of the catecholamines is to cause the bronchioles (air passages) in the lung to dilate. Blockage of these receptors in susceptible individuals (i.e., asthmatics) can lead to constriction of the bronchioles and a subsequent asthma attack. Since beta–1 selective beta–blockers such as metoprolol (Lopressor, Toprol XL) and atenolol (Tenormin) tend to bind strongly to the beta–1 receptors and only weakly to the beta–2 receptors, they tend to cause fewer asthma symptoms. Nonetheless, caution must be used when starting any person with asthma on any beta–blocker.

Beta–blockers not only block beta–receptors, but they also prevent the release of renin from the kidney. This in turn reduces the amount of angiotensin II circulating in the blood. Remember that angiotensin II is a very powerful vasoconstrictor of blood vessels, known to cause blood vessels to clamp down, which increases the blood pressure. Blocking the release of renin is therefore one additional way in which beta–blockers lower blood pressure. African Americans tend to have low levels of circulating renin (in other words, high renin level is not the cause of their high blood pressure), with the result that they have a less favorable response to beta–blockers than do whites. This, however, does not mean that they should not use them. An African American who has suffered a heart attack, for example, should certainly be treated with beta–blockers. Because the blood pressure–lowering effect of beta–blockers is enhanced by diuretics, and because it is known that African Americans typically respond well to diuretics, the combination of a diuretic and a beta-blocker (such as Ziac) is the logical choice for an African American who has both suffered a heart attack and has high blood pressure.

Other Uses

Beta-blockers are useful in a variety of conditions unrelated to high blood pressure and heart disease, including the treatment of migraine headaches, hand tremor, anxiety, stress, and hyperthyroidism. If you have one of these conditions as well as high blood pressure, your doctor might be able to treat both conditions with a single medication. In medical school one of my professors took his golf game very seriously. According to him, the secret of his success was taking a beta-blocker a few hours before a big match. His hands wouldn't shake, and he felt much calmer as he approached the green. I imagine this would be illegal in professional circles, but I can assure you he was an amateur golfer. I have often wondered what his non-physician golfing competitors would have said had they known about his self-medication with beta-blockers.

Finally, in the past beta-blockers were avoided by people with a history of congestive heart failure. The fear was that in this situation beta-blockers would slow down the heart rate and worsen the congestive heart failure. It turns out that often just the opposite is true. Although caution must be used in treating people with congestive heart failure with beta-blockers, in many cases, they improve the outcome of people with this condition.

Table 7.2 lists all currently available beta-blockers in the United States.

Since I think it is important to give diuretics in as low a dose as possible, the only combination beta-blocker/diuretic I routinely use is Ziac.

Table 7.2 Beta-Blockers and Dosages

BETA-BLOCKER	USUAL TOTAL DAILY DOSE (MG/DAY)	NUMBER OF DOSES PER DAY
Acebutolol (Sectral)[1]	200–800	1
Atenolol (Tenormin)[2]	25–100	2
Betaxolol (Kerlone)[2]	5–20	1
Bisprolol (Zebeta)[2]	2.5–10	1
Carteolol (Cartrol)	2.5–10	1
Carvedilol (Coreg)	2.5–50	2
Celiprolol (Selectol[2]	200–400	1
Labetalol (Normodyne, Trandate)	200–1200	2
Metoprolol (Lopressor,[2]	50–200	2
Toprol XL)[2]	50–200	1
Nadolol (Corgard)	40–320	1
Penbutolol (Levatol)	10–20	1
Pindolol (Visken)	10–60	2
Propranolol (Inderal,	40–480	2
Inderal LA)	40–480	1
Timolol (Blocadren)	20–60	2

Some preparations combine a beta-blocker with a diuretic:

Atenolol with Chlorthalidone (Tenoretic)	50/25–100/25	1
Bisoprolol with Hydrochlorothiazide (Ziac)	2.5/6.25–20/12.5	1
Lopressor with Hydrochlorothiazide (Lopressor HCT)	50/25–100/50	1–2

Table 7.2 continued

Propranolol with Hydrochlorothiazide (Inderide)	40/25–80/25	2
Propranolol with Hydrochlorothiazide (Inderide LA)	80/50–160/50	1
Timolol with Hydrochlorothiazide (Timolide)	10/25	2

[1]Moderate beta-1-Selectivity
[2]Significant beta-1-Selectivity

Which Beta-Blocker Is Right for You?

Once your doctor has decided that a beta-blocker is a good choice for you, she still has to decide which one of the many will be the best, given your particular circumstances. As a rule, all beta-blockers are equally effective in lowering blood pressure. However, there are still differences from one to another and these differences help predict their side effects. As mentioned earlier, one very important factor is the issue of beta-selectivity. The most beta-1-selective drugs (Tenormin, Kerlone, Zebeta, Selectral, Lopressor, and Toprol XL) would obviously be chosen for people with asthma who need a beta-blocker. Taking a beta-1-selective beta-blocker does not eliminate the risk of a medication-related asthma attack, but it does make it less likely.

Another reason to select a beta-1-selective beta-blocker is that they tend to have a less adverse effect on blood cholesterol and blood sugar levels than some nonselective agents. It is well known that beta-blockers have the potential to increase triglycerides (one of the blood fats—elevated levels increase the risk of heart disease and stroke) and lower HDL (the good cholesterol) levels.

Side Effects

Beta-blockers can raise blood sugar levels. In fact, a recent report from the Atherosclerosis Risk in Communities Study found that people with high blood pressure who were taking beta-blockers had a 28 percent greater risk of developing diabetes as compared to people with high blood pressure who were taking other types of blood pressure–lowering medications. Since the beta-1-selectives have less of a negative effect on triglycerides, HDL, and blood sugar, for people with these conditions they tend to be the best choice.

Another major side effect of the beta-blockers is the potential for causing sleep disturbances, nightmares, and vivid dreams. Beta-blockers can also make some people very tired and lethargic. Although any beta-blocker is capable of causing sleep disturbances and fatigue, the more lipid soluble it is, the more likely it is to get into the brain and cause these difficulties. Beta-blockers with the least lipid solubility include Tenormin, Kerlone, Cartrol, Selectol, and Corgard. Interestingly, the dream issue is a problem for some people but a blessing for others.

Just a few months ago Rose, an older woman who lives alone, was sent to see me because her triglycerides were 850 mg/dl (normal being less than 150 mg/dl). I noticed she was on Timolide (which is a combination of timolol—a nonbeta-1-selective but highly lipid soluble beta-blocker—and hydrochlorothiazide). She had been treating her high blood pressure by taking Timolide twice a day for about two years. She was also taking oral estrogen, and had done so since she had had a hysterectomy about ten years earlier.

When I see a person for high triglycerides my first task is to determine if I might be able to lower her triglycerides into the normal range (below 150 mg/dl) without the use of a triglyceride-lowering medication. The currently available triglyceride-lowering medications (Niaspan, Tricor, Lopid) are all excellent drugs, but if I can manage without adding a medication I do so.

In Rose's case, components of both the Timolide and the oral estrogen were causing her triglycerides to rise. I called her doctor to ask if there was a special reason that he had chosen Timolide for her. He said he had actually chosen it because he happened to have samples of it in his office and as it worked well, he left her on it. With regard to the estrogen, I asked if he would have any objections if I switched Rose to the transdermal estrogen. I explained that the transdermal estrogen (applied to the skin as a patch) does not cause the same undesirable effects on the triglycerides as does the oral estrogen. In both cases, he agreed to switch Rose to more "triglyceride friendly" medications. I told Rose that rather than adding a medication to treat her triglycerides, what I wanted to do was taper off her Timolide and take her off her oral estrogen. In both cases she would require a replacement. I explained that tapering her off the Timolide was essential to prevent a dramatic rise in her blood pressure.

When I saw she was a little reluctant to change the Timolide, which was, after all, controlling her blood pressure beautifully, I told her that she might actually feel better not taking it. I explained that one of the side effects of beta-blockers could be bad dreams or very vivid dreams. Her reaction was one I never expected: She told me she didn't know whether to laugh or cry. Since she had been on the Timolide she had had a recurrent dream of a large, very frightening woman with long dark hair, who would appear at her bedside menacingly, muttering unintelligible threats. Rose told me that the dreams began just around the time she went on the Timolide. She had never told her children because she was afraid they would think she was crazy. She told me that she would have the dream about once a week and was then unable to get back to sleep.

I told her I couldn't promise the Timolide was the cause but it was certainly a possibility. I switched Rose to amlodipine (Norvasc), a long-acting calcium channel blocker. This once-a-day drug has no effect on triglycerides, tends to be quite effective in older people, and does not cause bad dreams.

I also asked her if she would object to switching the way she took her estrogen. I told her she would be getting the same drug but instead of taking it by mouth, which tends to raise triglycerides, she would use an estrogen patch, which would deliver it through her skin. She would need to change the patch once a week. Her only concern was whether she could shower with it on. When I said that was not a problem, she agreed to the switch.

Finally I explained that lifestyle changes could have a profound impact on both blood pressure and triglycerides. It turned out that Rose was routinely having two glasses of sherry each evening (to help her sleep), she had no regular exercise routine, and she needed to lose about 25 pounds.

Rose agreed to limit her sherry intake to three drinks a week, and she made some dramatic improvements in her diet. She increased her intake of potassium-rich foods because this can improve blood pressure, and she cut calories (particularly sugar calories, which tend to result in triglyceride increases). Finally, because of her age, I asked her to undergo a stress test prior to beginning a daily walking program. After she passed with flying colors, I asked her to gradually build up to walking three miles a day. I explained that for her, exercise would have many benefits: It would lower triglycerides, blood pressure, and weight and would likely improve her sleep patterns. Finally, women who exercise are about 50 percent less likely to die of heart disease than women who are sedentary.

Eight weeks later Rose had lost 10 pounds, her triglycerides were 132 mg/dl, her blood pressure was a perfect 130/78 mmHg, and best of all, she had not had any more bad dreams.

On the other hand, some people truly enjoy the vivid dreams. George is a science fiction writer. I put him on Toprol XL about three years ago after his heart attack. Prior to the attack he had been struggling with writer's block. In fact, he had missed a major deadline with his publisher; but because of his condition, the publisher was understanding and gave him an extension. When I saw him about ten weeks after the heart attack, I asked if the Toprol was causing any side effects. "Such as what?" he wanted to know. I told him that the beta-blockers could cause sleep disturbances, vivid dreams, nightmares, fatigue, and sometimes even impotence.

He practically kissed me. "So you are responsible for the end of my writer's block!" he said, sounding delighted. He told me he was not fatigued and his sex life was great. But ever since his heart attack he was having the most amazing dreams. He had taken to leaving a pen and pad by his bedside so that he could jot down the dream the moment he woke up—he had already incorporated many of the ideas into his new science fiction novel. He told me that if he had been placed on beta-blockers twenty years ago he probably would have been more successful than Stephen King.

It is amazing to me how the same side effect can be so troublesome to one person and such a blessing to another.

The issue of impotence is a serious one for some men who take beta-blockers. In the Medical Research Council (MRC) Trial, a study of more than seventeen thousand people (52 percent male), 13.2 percent of those on the beta-blocker propranolol complained of impotence, while only 10.1 percent of those on placebo had this complaint. Impotence can occur with any of the beta-blockers. Your doctor may fail to ask if you are having a problem. If you are, do not hesitate to discuss this. Even though beta-blockers can prolong life after a heart attack, for some people this side effect is unacceptable.

Len is a patient I have been seeing for over five years. He was referred to me just after his heart attack. I put him a beta-blocker and, luckily, remembered to ask him about impotence. He told me he didn't care if the beta-blocker lengthened his life—that "the way I am feeling right now, no matter how long I get, it will seem like too long." I got the point. I switched him to the calcium channel blocker Norvasc to control his angina, and he has been much happier ever since.

All beta-blockers can lead to reductions in exercise tolerance. Although this can present a major problem for some people, most can develop an exercise program and achieve cardiovascular fitness while on a beta-blocker.

Finally, it is important to note once again that beta-blockers can protect against the recurrence of heart disease. Unless there is a very good reason not to, if you have heart disease, you should be on a beta-blocker!

CALCIUM CHANNEL BLOCKERS

In the early 1980s calcium channel blockers (CCBs) began to be widely used for the management of high blood pressure. There are two different groups of calcium channel blockers: the dihydropyridines and the nondihydropyridines. The calcium channel blockers work by blocking the ability of calcium to enter the cells of the blood vessels, resulting in vasodilatation (opening up) of the blood vessels and a drop in blood pressure.

Although all the CCBs dilate the heart arteries to some degree, it appears that the dihydropyridines may have the greatest impact on these particular blood vessels. When the heart arteries are dilated, blood flow to the heart is increased. This effect of the dihydropyridines make them particularly useful in treating angina—chest pain caused by a reduction in blood flow to the heart, generally as a result of cholesterol blockages in the arteries.

All calcium channel blockers prevent calcium from entering the cells and hence cause vasodilatation, but the two classes of CCBs are chemically different. Even within the nondihydropyridine group, diltiazem and verapamil have significant differences in chemical structure and in their side effects. Table 7.3 lists the currently available CCBs, their usual daily dosages, and how frequently they must be taken. Table 7.4 lists their most common side effects.

Table 7.3 Calcium Channel Blockers and Dosages

CCB CLASS	TRADE NAME	USUAL TOTAL DAILY DOSAGE (MG/DAY)	NUMBER OF DOSES/DAY
Dihydropyridines			
Amlodipine	Norvasc	2.5–10	1
Felodipine	Plendil	2.5–20	1
Isradipine	DynaCirc	5–20	2
DynaCirc CR	DynaCirc CR	5–20	1
Nicardipine	Cardene SR	60–90	2
Nifedipine	Procardia XL, Adalat	30–120	1
Nisoldipine	Sular	20–60	1
Nondihydropyridines			
Verapamil	Isoptin SR, Calan SR	90–480	2
	Verelan, Covera HS	120–480	1
Diltiazem	Cardizem SR	120–360	2
	Cardizem CD, Dilacor XR, Tiazac	120–360	1

Table 7.4 Side Effects of Calcium Channel Blockers

SIDE EFFECT	DIHYDROPYRIDINES	NONDIHYDROPYRIDINES	
		VERAPAMIL	DILTIAZEM
Sudden/rapid drop in blood pressure	++	+	+
Flushing	++	+	−
Headache	++	+	+
Fluid in ankles[1]	++	+	+
Used to treat heart arrhythmias	−	++	+
Slow pulse rate	−	++	+
Increase pulse rate[2]	+	−	−
Constipation	−	++	+
Gum tissue overgrowth[3]	++	+	+
Increase in nighttime urination	+	+	+/−
Reduce second heart attack	−	+	−
Reduce mortality after heart attack	−	+	−
Prevent stroke in the elderly[4]	+	−	−

[1]Fluid in ankles can be dramatically reduced by adding an ACE inhibitor.
[2]The dihydropyridines tend to increase heart rate when first begun but pulse rate quickly returns to pretreatment level. The one exception is with nifedipine where pulse rate can increase and remain elevated.
[3]Gum tissue overgrowth, or enlargement of gums, is frequently noted by dentists.
[4]Stroke reduced in the Syst-Eur (European Trial of Systemic Hypertension in the Elderly) by 42 percent. In this same trial, cardiac events were reduced by 26 percent in patients receiving the dihydropyridine Nitrendipine. At this time Nitrendipine is not available in the United States.

Differences from Other Blood Pressure Medications

Unlike the blood pressure medications we have discussed thus far in this chapter (diuretics and beta-blockers), neither the dihydropyridines or the nondihydropyridines have an adverse effect on blood cholesterol, blood sugar, blood potassium, or uric acid levels. Of course, they do have the side effects listed in Table 7.4, but as a rule they are very well tolerated.

It is also important to mention that, unlike most other classes of blood pressure–lowering medications, the blood pressure–lowering effect of all CCBs is usually not reduced in people who are also taking nonsteroidal anti-inflammatory drugs such as Motrin or Naproxin. This is an important point because many people have both high blood pressure and arthritis or other chronic conditions requiring daily use of these nonsteroidal medications. The side effects listed for the dihydropyridines are most pronounced for nifedipine. Newer dihydropyridines such as Norvasc and even long-acting nifedipine are much less troublesome.

Calcium Channel Blockers and Grapefruit Juice

About a year or so ago, a great deal of press was given to the fact that drinking grapefruit juice could increase blood levels of the dihydropyridines. Although this does seem to be true for felodipine (Plendil) and nifedipine (Procardia XL, Adalat), it does not hold true for amlodipine (Norvasc).

I am convinced that too much was made of this finding. However, just to be on the safe side, if you are on Plendil, Procardia XL, or Adalat, I recommend drinking orange juice as opposed to grapefruit juice. You might be saying to yourself, if I have high blood pressure, what could be the problem with drinking grapefruit juice to lower my pressure further? The concern is that once your blood pressure is well controlled with a CCB, the addition of large amounts of grapefruit juice might drop your blood pressure so low that you would faint.

Interactions with Other Drugs and Other Side Effects

As a group the CCBs have relatively few interactions with other drugs, but there are some that you should be aware of. Table 7.5 lists the drug interactions that have been reported for both classes of CCBs. These interactions apply generally to all CCBs. Each group has its own characteristics, however, and must be considered separately as well.

As you can see from the previous tables, there are now a large number of dihydropyridines. Nifedipine was the prototype and was originally available only in a rapidly acting capsule form. This early formulation acted in minutes to dilate blood vessels and dramatically lower blood pressure. Unfortunately the blood vessels to the brain as well as to the skin were markedly affected, with the predictable side effects of headache, dizziness, and flushing.

When I was working in the medical intensive care unit at the University of Massachusetts Medical Center, I treated a man whose blood pressure was 210/110 mmHg with short-acting nifedipine. Within minutes his blood pressure was 110/60 mmHg, but he was dizzy, flushed, and had a headache, and he told me with firm conviction that my cure was worse than his disease. Fortunately for patients, only rarely is the short-acting nifedipine ever needed. My patient did very well, but I could tell he never liked me very much. Since the dark ages of my residency, the short-acting nifedipine has been replaced by the long-acting preparations Procardia XL and Adalat. Although these preparations can cause the same side effects, they occur less frequently.

I frequently prescribe the dihydropyridine amlodipine (Norvasc). I am particularly pleased with the fact that even though it is taken only once a day, it actually has an even longer impact on blood pressure. In fact, you could forget to take it on a given day and your blood pressure will probably still be well controlled. Because studies have shown that many people do indeed forget at least one dose a week, this feature is particularly attractive!

Table 7.5 Drug–Drug Interactions with Calcium Channel Blockers

CCB	INTERACTING MEDICATION	RESULT
Dihydropyridines and nondihydropyridines	Cyclosporin[1]	Elevated blood cyclosporin level
Dihydropridines and nondihydropyridines	Cimetidine[2]	Elevated blood CCB level
Dihydropyridines	Propranolol[3]	Elevated blood propranolol level
Verapamil	Beta-blockers	Excessive reduction in pulse
		Excessive reduction in blood pressure
		Dramatic reduction in heart rate
Verapamil	Digoxin[4]	Elevated blood digoxin level

[1]**Cyclosporin is an immunosuppressive agent used by people who have had organ transplants.**
[2]**Cimetidine is used to control excess stomach acid.**
[3]**Propranolol is a beta-blocker used to control blood pressure.**
[4]**Digoxin is a medication used to control heart rate.**

One of the most common side effects seen with Norvasc is ankle edema (fluid). Many people try to treat this with a diuretic; however, because this excess fluid is unrelated to water retention, diuretics do not help at all. Rather, it is believed that this side effect is related to the fact that dihydropyridines such as Norvasc dilate arteries more than veins. Some studies have found that the addition of an ACE inhibitor, probably because they dilate veins, helps prevent this unpleasant side effect.

You might guess from the previous table that your doctor would be likely to consider using a dihydropyridine to treat your high blood pressure if you have diabetes or high cholesterol. In both of these situations, dihydropyridines have no adverse impact on blood sugar or cholesterol level. People with gout (a painful disorder characterized by painful, swollen red joints, especially in the great toe) caused by elevated uric acid levels do well on any CCB, including the dihydropyridines.

People who require nonsteroidal anti–inflammatory medications for the treatment of arthritic conditions or other muscle or joint problems also do well on the dihydropyridines. Some studies have shown that people who find it difficult to give up a high-salt diet still respond well to the dihydropyridines. Although I certainly do not recommend that my patients continue eating excessive salt, many other blood pressure medications just can't work well in the face of a high-salt diet.

In addition, nifedipine has been shown to be useful in stalling the need for aortic valve replacement in people who suffer from a leaky aortic valve. This is especially important for people who are at high risk of a poor surgical outcome.

Finally, if you have had a stroke or a heart attack, a drug in this class might be considered. Data from the Syst-Eur Trial (European Trial of Systemic Hypertension in the Elderly) found that patients receiving the dihydropyridine Nitrendipine suffered 42 percent fewer strokes, while cardiac events were reduced by 26 percent. At this time Nitrendipine is not available in the United States, but in my opinion, other dihydropyridines are also likely to be protective.

Nondihydropyridines

The nondihydropyridines verapamil and diltiazem require a separate discussion. In the 1960s an intravenous form of verapamil was used to treat heart arrhythmias. The heart arrhythmias verapamil worked best on were those related to rapid heart rate such as atrial fibrillation (a heart arrhythmia in which the top chambers of the heart beat as fast as 400–600 beats per minute). Since verapamil is so effective at slowing the heart rate, you might guess that it could also be too efficient.

This is true. In the past, when verapamil was sometimes paired with a beta-blocker (remember that beta-blockers can slow the heart rate too), the consequence for some people was complete heart block. The top part of your heart consists of two atria and the bottom of two ventricles. A group of specialized cells in the right atrium sends electrical impulses to the cells of both ventricles. These impulses signal the ventricle to contract and make the heart beat. The combination of verapamil and a beta-blocker can poison the transmission of these electrical impulses. The result is that the ventricles can continue to beat, but at an extremely slow rate.

Fainting is the simplest consequence. For some individuals, the combination can be life threatening. For this reason, with very few exceptions, verapamil should never be paired with a beta-blocker.

Since verapamil has been clearly shown to decrease the risk of a second heart attack and also has been shown to decrease mortality following a heart attack, if a beta-blocker cannot be used following a heart attack, then verapamil should be instituted. As you remember, beta-blockers are the first choice drug following a heart attack; however, in certain people (for example, asthmatics or people who have unacceptable side effects while on beta-blockers) they cannot be used. In such situations verapamil is a logical choice.

The CONVINCE Trial

At the New England Heart Institute where I work, we are currently involved in a five-year study called the CONVINCE trial. This study is designed to compare the outcomes (in terms of heart disease events and stroke) of people with high blood pressure who are treated with either Covera HS (a long-acting form of verapamil) or atenolol (a beta-blocker). Many, but not all, of the study participants have already suffered a heart attack or stroke.

Covera HS is a specially designed capsule preparation of verapamil, which is taken at bedtime. The medication is released so that peak levels of the drug are achieved in the early morning hours. There is an excellent theoretical reason for this design: It is well known that blood pressure peaks at this time and is associated with an increase in heart attacks. It is hoped that this preparation will result in a substantial reduction in heart and stroke risk.

To date (the trial is in its third year) we have been impressed with how well our patients have done. Some of our participants have complained of constipation, which is in fact the most common complaint of people on verapamil. This problem can generally be managed by increasing dietary fiber and water. We have, however, had a few people drop out of the study because of this consequence.

Diltiazem appears to have side effects that lie in between those of the dihydropyridines and verapamil. Although diltiazem can cause flushing, dizziness, and leg edema, it appears to do so less frequently than the dihydropyridines. And although it has been associated with slowing of the heart rate and constipation, the impact is less dramatic than seen with verapamil.

Since the dihydropyridines and nondihydropyridines have different chemical structures, Saseen and colleagues wondered if it might be possible to combine these two groups of CCBs and get an additive effect on blood pressure reduction. The answer was yes. If a dihydropyridine works well for you but fails to fully normalize your blood pressure, don't be surprised if your doctor adds a nondihydropyridine to your therapy.

In the past there was a general opinion in the medical community that older people responded better to CCBs than did younger people. As further studies have been performed, this finding has not been borne out. It is now clear that all ages and all races respond equally well to this group of medications.

Other Uses

Very preliminary data suggest that CCBs may be beneficial in the treatment of a wide variety of medical conditions including migraine headaches, Raynaud's disease (a circulatory disorder), nighttime leg cramps, asthma, Alzheimer's disease, and even epilepsy. At this point it is premature to initiate the CCBs to treat the aforementioned conditions and diseases, but as more evidence becomes available the CCBs may be appealing blood pressure–lowering medications for people who have high blood pressure and one of these additional conditions.

In my experience, the CCBs work beautifully for the control of Raynaud's disease. Mr. Doherty, one of my patients, had been on amlodipine (Norvasc) as a blood pressure–lowering medication for years. As far as he was concerned, the only reason he was taking Norvasc was to control his high blood pressure. When I first met him he was 15 pounds overweight and was interested in coming off his blood pressure–lowering medication. After he lost the 15 pounds and his blood pressure dropped from 138/80 mmHg to 110/60 mmHg, I told him he had earned the right to see if it would stay down without the Norvasc.

He left my office feeling so pleased with himself. I asked him to return in one month to reassess his blood pressure. He agreed to check his pressure at home on his reliable home monitor and to call me if he noted a significant rise. Almost immediately after coming off the Norvasc he began to experience severe symptoms of Raynaud's.

When he walked outside to get the paper two days after stopping the Norvasc, his fingers became white and painful. When he went back indoors, they first turned blue and then, rewarming, they became red and throbbing. The entire experience recurred several times before he called and asked if this might have anything to do with coming off the Norvasc. Since he was not planning to move away from New England, he is back on his Norvasc but recognizes that now he is treating Raynaud's disease, not high blood pressure. Other CCBs such as diltiazem and nifedipine are also used to treat this condition.

CCBs and the Risk of Heart Attack and Cancer

A last word on CCBs. You may remember a 1995 study (it got a lot of media attention) suggesting a link between the short-acting forms of the CCBs and the development of heart attack. A more recent study suggested that in the elderly, the use of short-acting CCBs might increase the risk of cancer. Although these studies have not been substantiated, they cannot simply be dismissed.

The most important thing to understand is that these studies are based on the use of short-acting CCBs, which are almost never used in clinical practice. The short-acting CCBs, which must be taken two to three times a day, have now been almost completely replaced by long-acting (once a day) forms of these same medications.

The difference between the two formulations is significant. Because the short-acting CCBs are taken at intervals throughout the day, the result is large swings in their concentration in the patient's blood. Many scientists feel that it is the high (peak) blood levels of these medications that increase the risk of complications. The long-acting forms of CCBs behave quite differently, since they are formulated for a slow and steady release of medication and provide more consistent blood levels and better blood pressure control.

With regard to the issue of cancer, there was no consistent trend as to the type of cancer involved. Although the elderly patients on short-acting CCBs had a slight increase in a wide variety of cancers, no one type emerged as being causally related. Since cancers in various organs have very different causes, the lack of an increase in a specific cancer weakens the case considerably.

In the next five years, we will have the results of a multitude of studies being conducted in Europe and the United States. These studies will compare long-acting CCBs with other antihypertensive medications in very large numbers of patients. Many of these studies have been ongoing for at least four to five years and none have been halted early due to side effects of the long-acting CCBs. Although these studies are typically blind (meaning neither the physician nor the patient knows which medication is being taken), there is always an oversight board for any large study. This group is responsible for reviewing all side effects of the study medications. They are legally and morally bound to halt a study if one class of drugs is either dramatically worse or better than the other drugs being observed.

Mark, a forty-five-year-old machine shop supervisor, was sent to me because his doctor was concerned that despite taking verapamil at 120 mg three times a day, his blood pressure was not well controlled. I saw him at 4:00 P.M. on a Tuesday afternoon. He had come straight from work and his blood pressure was 166/105 mmHg. I asked him when his last dose of verapamil had been, and he told me that it had been some time the day before. As he put it himself, "I can't remember a medication more than once a day."

Since he was tolerating the verapamil well (when he remembered to take it), I switched him to Covera HS (a long-acting form of verapamil) at 240 mg per night. He returned one week later with a blood pressure of 136/82 mmHg. Clearly he was responsive to the drug. I hate to think of the swings in his pressure prior to switching to the once-a-day preparation.

ANGIOTENSIN-CONVERTING ENZYME INHIBITORS

Angiotensin-converting enzyme inhibitors (ACE inhibitors, for short) are among the best-tolerated blood pressure–lowering medications available. The first ACE inhibitor was derived from the venom of a Brazilian snake. It required an injection and was never used in humans. But it wasn't long before an oral version was developed.

The first ACE inhibitor to be routinely used in the United States was captopril (Capoten). Initially it was reserved for people with very severe high blood pressure. This was because the use of Capoten was associated with significant and potentially life-threatening hypotension (low blood pressure). It turned out that the main reason for this side effect was that early on Capoten was used in extraordinarily high doses (sometimes as much as 300 mg three times a day). Once it was determined that as little as 12.5 mg three times a day was often sufficient to normalize blood pressure, Capoten was ready for prime time. Because it is difficult for most people to remember to take any drug three times a day, 25 mg twice a day has also been shown to be effective.

How They Work

All ACE inhibitors work by preventing the conversion of angiotensin I (AI) to angiotensin II (AII). Angiotensin II (as noted in chapter 2) is one of the most potent vasoconstrictors known. A vasoconstrictor is a substance that can cause the body's arteries to clamp down, which in turn results in a marked increase in blood pressure. There is no doubt that the ACE inhibitors have a multitude of other effects—one is preventing the breakdown of bradykinin, a substance in the blood that dilates blood vessels and leads to a reduction in blood pressure. Table 7.6 lists all of the currently available ACE inhibitors.

Who Should Take an ACE Inhibitor

As I try to decide if an ACE inhibitor would be a good choice as a medication, I consider a person's cardiac status. ACE inhibitors are

Table 7.6 ACE Inhibitors

ACE INHIBITORS	USUAL TOTAL DOSE (MG/DAY)	NUMBER OF DOSES/DAY
Benazepril (Lotensin)	10–40	1
Captopril (Capoten)	25–150	2–3
Enalapril (Vasotec)	5–40	2
Fosinopril (Monopril)	10–40	1
Lisinopril (Prinivil, Zestril)	5–40	1
Moexipril (Univasc)	25–100	2
Quinapril (Accupril)	5–80	1
Ramipril (Altace)	1.25–20	1
Trandolapril (Mavik)[1]	1–4	1[1]

[1]**Trandolapril (Mavik) has a greater than 24-hour effect. As a result, for many people blood pressure remains well controlled even if they miss a dose of the medication.**

especially useful blood pressure–lowering agents in people with depressed heart function. Because a heart attack damages the heart muscle, many people are left with an organ that doesn't pump as well as it did prior to the attack. In this situation, the use of ACE inhibitors has been found to decrease mortality and so should be used. In fact, given these circumstances, I use them even in people who do not have high blood pressure.

In addition to their beneficial cardiac effects, ACE inhibitors are known to improve a person's ability to respond to insulin. Insulin, a hormone made by the pancreas, is responsible for promoting the efficient removal of sugar from the blood. If you have diabetes, you may be able to reduce your dose of insulin or other diabetes medication after being started on an ACE inhibitor. Likewise, if your diabetes has been well controlled on the same dose of medication for a prolonged time, you may suddenly experience a significant drop in your blood sugar with the initiation of an ACE inhibitor. This should not be considered a reason to avoid them, however. On the contrary, ACE inhibitors are considered to be the ideal choice for people with diabetes. You should, however, check your blood sugar more frequently when beginning an ACE inhibitor, because you may need a lower dose of your diabetes medication.

Aside from improving blood sugar, the ACE inhibitors are considered the drug of choice for diabetics with high blood pressure because this class of medications has been shown to protect kidney function. The importance of this cannot be stressed enough. Diabetes is the most common cause of renal (kidney) failure in this country. So as a rule, ACE inhibitors are the ideal drugs for people with high blood pressure and kidney disease. One of the early signs of kidney disease is the appearance of protein in the urine. The ACE inhibitors dramatically reduce this.

There is one exception to this rule. Some people have reduced kidney function because of blockages in their kidney arteries. These blockages can be caused by either cholesterol (this tends to occur most commonly in smokers with high cholesterol) or by thickening of the muscular layers of the arteries leading to the kidney. This is called fibromuscular dysplasia. It occurs primarily in young women and may be the cause of the sudden appearance of high blood pressure in a woman who previously had normal or low blood pressure.

In both of these situations starting an ACE inhibitor will reduce blood pressure beautifully but will also lead to a further reduction in blood flow through the diseased kidney arteries. The end result is worsening kidney function. In fact, in the past captopril was sometimes given to people suspected of having a blockage in the kidney arteries as a way to diagnose kidney disease. This was called the "Captopril Challenge Test."

As your doctor decides if you are likely to respond favorably to an ACE inhibitor she will take into account your race. Caucasians tend to respond better to ACE inhibitors than do African Americans. Unlike some other classes of medication, the young and the old respond equally well.

Combinations with Other Blood Pressure Medications

ACE inhibitors are very versatile and can be paired with other blood pressure–lowering medications including the calcium channel blockers (CCBs) and diuretics (with the exception of potassium sparing diuretics—see below). Like CCBs, the ACE inhibitors do not have a negative effect on cholesterol or blood sugar levels. (In fact as mentioned, blood sugar may fall.)

Side Effects

It is important to mention that ACE inhibitors can lead to an increase in blood potassium levels. Although this is rarely cause for concern, as the potassium level increases only slightly, in some cases, especially if a potassium–sparing diuretic is also being taken, a person can develop a dangerously high level.

The most common side effects of the ACE inhibitors are a dry hacking cough and bronchospasm (constriction of the small tubules leading to the lung). The cough may begin when the ACE inhibitor is first started or it can develop even months after starting it. It appears that the cough is much more common in women, African Americans, and in up to 50 percent of Chinese patients started on ACE inhibitors. As a rule, the cough subsides within a few weeks of stopping the drug and returns immediately if it is restarted.

Although very rare, the most severe side effect that can occur with the use of an ACE inhibitor is angioedema (occurring in about one per thousand people). Angioedema is swelling of the deep layers of the skin and mucosal surfaces of the throat and mouth (although swelling can occur almost anywhere, including the arms, face, lips, and throat.) Because swelling of throat tissue could prevent a person from breathing, this can be a life-threatening complication. In general angioedema occurs with a person's first dose of an ACE inhibitor.

Typically the swelling is easily treated with either Benadryl or steroids. Since it is impossible to predict who will develop this potentially fatal side effect, it is important that you be aware of it. I recommend having a supply of Benadryl available when you take your first dose, as well as being sure you take your first dose at a time when you are not alone.

After making these suggestions for years to patients who never needed them, I recently had my first patient who did.

I was at home with my children on my day off when my secretary, Diane, called to tell me she had just gotten a call from Mrs. Richards, a woman I had seen the day before and started on an ACE inhibitor. Diane said Mrs. Richards was having trouble breathing and that her lips were swelling. I knew right away what was going on.

I called her and instructed her to take two Benadryl. She was able to speak to me, so I knew she was still breathing without too much effort. Nonetheless, I told her I would like to call an ambulance to bring her to the emergency room where she would be able to receive intravenous medications if necessary. She declined the ambulance, saying that her husband would drive her in. By the time she arrived in the emergency room she was breathing easily but her lips were still swollen. Needless to say, she won't be taking an ACE inhibitor again. This is a very rare side effect, but one that must always be kept in mind.

Capoten, more than the other ACE inhibitors, has been reported to occasionally cause a variety of side effects, including a metallic taste. This unpleasant side effect is generally, but not always, transient. Capoten has also been reported to cause an itchy rash and at times can cause significant reduction in white blood cell count.

ACE Inhibitors and Pregnancy

Under no circumstances should ACE inhibitors be given to a pregnant woman because they can cause fetal death. It is my practice not to prescribe ACE inhibitors to young women who have the potential to become pregnant unless they are using a reliable form of birth control. It is reassuring, however, that many healthy babies have been born to women who were on ACE inhibitors, but who stopped very early in their pregnancies. Nonetheless, given the fact that there are many other blood pressure–lowering medications available, I do not think the benefits of ACE inhibitors outweigh the risks for a woman who might become pregnant. There are many other excellent and safe choices for a pregnant woman with high blood pressure.

Heart Disease

One of the most recent ACE inhibitors trials published is the HOPE (Heart Outcomes Preventive Evaluation) Trial. It found that even in people without high blood pressure, the ACE inhibitor ramipril (Altace) dramatically reduced the risk of heart attacks, strokes, or death in individuals at high risk of heart disease. These people did not have evidence of heart failure. This is important because since the ACE inhibitors have already been shown to benefit people with heart failure, the HOPE trial extends the number of people who can benefit from this medication.

ANGIOTENSIN-RECEPTOR ANTAGONISTS (SARTANS)

Very recently a new family of blood pressure medications called angiotensin-receptor antagonists (sartans) was developed. They also work on the renin–angiotensin system. But unlike the ACE inhibitors, which prevent angiotensin II from being formed, this class of drugs works by preventing angiotensin II from attaching to its receptor on the blood vessel. By preventing this action the sartans prevent the constriction (and high blood pressure) caused by angiotensin II.

Because this class of drugs is very new, there have been few clinical trials comparing them to other blood pressure–lowering medications. One relatively small trial that has been completed is the ELITE trial. This trial compared losartan (Cozaar), the first sartan to come on the market, to captopril (Capoten), an ACE inhibitor. (See previous section.) The 722 patients who participated in the trial didn't necessarily all have high blood pressure; however, all participants were over sixty-five and all had heart failure.

Losartan (Cozaar) lowered mortality significantly more than did captopril (Capoten). In the ELITE trial, while death occurred in a substantial number of the Cozaar-treated group (4.8 percent), a much larger percentage of the Capoten treated group died (8.7 percent). The significant number of deaths in each group confirms that people over sixty-five who have congestive heart failure are a high-risk group. In this study it appeared that Cozaar may afford more protection than Capoten. The study investigators are continuing this trial with over three thousand patients to determine if there really is a survival advantage with Cozaar as compared to Capoten.

Who Might Benefit

Why might your doctor prescribe a sartan for you? They have been shown to be as effective in lowering blood pressure as most other antihypertensive agents, but they also appear to have very few side effects. They seem to be equally effective in men and women, and the young and the old benefit equally. It has, however, been noted that while responsive to the sartans, African Americans generally require somewhat higher doses to achieve a satisfactory effect. Table 7.7 lists the sartans currently available.

Side Effects

This class of drugs has had few reported side effects. They are a nice alternative to ACE inhibitors for people who have been trou-

Table 7.7 Angiotensin–Receptor Antagonists (Sartans)

SARTAN	USUAL TOTAL DAILY DOSE (MG/DAY)	NUMBER OF DOSES/DAY
Losartan (Cozaar)	25–100	1–2
Valsartan (Diovan)	80–320	1
Irbesartan (Avapro)	150–300	1

bled by cough, which has not been reported with the sartans. Like the ACE inhibitors, they protect kidney function and reduce the loss of protein from the kidney in people who already have kidney problems.

Like the ACE inhibitors, sartans lower blood pressure but cause deteriorating kidney function in people with blockages in their kidney arteries. This class of drugs should be avoided during pregnancy. Finally, sartans can sometimes increase blood potassium levels, and although rare, angioedema can occur with the sartans as it can with the ACE inhibitors.

Prior to Cozaar coming on the market, my department at the New England Heart Institute in Manchester, NH participated in a trial using this agent. Of the large number of patients we enrolled, not a single one experienced a drug-related side effect. Since that time I have prescribed all of the sartans, and I have been thrilled with their performance. I have had some patients for whom the sartans did not do the entire job, and in these situations I have added a small dose of a diuretic with great success.

In fact, all three sartans are available in combination with hydrochlorothiazide. Hyzaar contains 50 mg of losartan paired with 12.5 mg of hydrochlorothiazide. Avalide comes in two strengths: 150 mg or 300 mg of irbesartan in combination with 12.5 mg of hydrochlorothiazide. Diovan HCT is the combination of valsartan and 12.5 mg of hydrochlorothiazide.

ALPHA–ADRENERGIC BLOCKERS

Alpha-adrenergic blockers, not surprisingly, block the alpha receptors on blood vessels. The result of this action is that norepinephrine, which normally attaches to the alpha receptor, is no longer able to do its job. As mentioned earlier, norepinephrine is a chemical released into the blood at nerve endings. When norepinephrine attaches to the alpha-adrenergic receptors on the body's blood vessels, it sends a signal to the vessels telling them to constrict. This action leads to an increase in blood pressure; blocking it causes the vessels to dilate. In the past I have frequently prescribed alpha-blockers because they not only improve blood pressure, but also effect positive metabolic changes such as improving cholesterol and fasting insulin levels.

The ALLHAT Trial

My use of alpha-blockers has been dramatically altered by the data released on March 8, 2000 by ALLHAT (Antihypertensive and Lipid Lowering Treatment to Prevent Heart Attack Trial). ALLHAT is a National Institutes of Health–sponsored trial that involves 42,448 patients being treated at 623 clinics throughout North America. ALLHAT, which began in 1994, is comparing chlorthaledone (a diuretic), doxazosin (an alpha-blocker), amlodipine (a calcium channel blocker), and lisinopril (an angiotensin-converting enzyme inhibitor).

As with any large-scale clinical trial, data from ALLHAT have been continuously reviewed by an independent data review and advisory board. In early March, 2000 the board recommended halting the alpha-blocker arm of the study. People randomized to doxazosin (also known as Cardura) were found to have 25 percent more cardiovascular events and were twice as likely to be hospitalized for congestive heart failure as were people in the chlorthaledone (diuretic) arm of the trial. Participants in the alpha-blocker arm of the trial were encouraged to stay in the trial but their medication was changed to one of the other study drugs.

The findings from ALLHAT came as a surprise to everyone involved. They underscore the importance of clinical trials.

At any given time, the average physician has between fifteen hundred to twenty-five hundred people under his care. While this may seem like a large number of people, it took a study of forty-two thousand people to discover that alpha-blockers are not as good as diuretics. They lower blood pressure just as well as diuretics, but the side effect profile is considerably worse.

If you are on one of the currently available alpha-blockers (terazosin marketed as Hytrin, prazosin marketed as Minipress, or doxazosin, the agent used in ALLHAT and marketed as Cardura), it is crucial that you consult your physician before going off the medication.

When to Use

Although the alpha-blockers are surely no longer recommended as a first-line medication for the treatment of hypertension, they may be appropriate as second- or third-line drugs. As a class they do have some important side benefits.

Prostate Enlargement

All alpha-blockers have been shown to decrease the symptoms of benign prostatic hypertrophy (BPH). As men age, they almost invariably begin to have some enlargement of the prostate gland. This results in obstruction to urinary flow, and the end result is frequent urination, especially at night. Some men report needing to get up to urinate three or four times in a night. The discovery that the alpha-adrenergic blockers could dramatically and quickly improve symptoms and often prevent or delay surgery for this condition has suddenly improved the popularity of these agents.

Table 7.8 Alpha-Adrenergic Blockers

ALPHA-ADRENERGIC BLOCKER	USUAL TOTAL DAILY DOSE (MG/DAY)	NUMBER OF DOSES/DAY
Doxazosin (Cardura)	1–16	1
Prazosin (Minipress)	2–30	2
Terazosin (Hytrin)	1–20	1

Two additional alpha-adrenergic blockers are available in the United States: phenoxybenzamine and phentolamine. These drugs are used exclusively in the treatment of pheochromocytoma, a rare disease that causes marked elevations in blood pressure. See chapter 9.

Other Side Effects and Benefits

Table 7.8 lists the currently available alpha-adrenergic blockers. Overall the alpha-adrenergic blockers are well tolerated. The most common side effect tends to be dizziness, which for most people is only transient. If your doctor prescribes an alpha-blocker (say as a second agent), you should be sure to take the first dose at night and use great caution if a trip to the bathroom is necessary. Alpha-blockers can improve cholesterol and fasting insulin levels. Since high blood pressure is often found in people with high cholesterol and/or diabetes, this side benefit may be important for some people. Most studies have found a reduction in LDL-cholesterol (low-density lipoprotein cholesterol, also known as the bad cholesterol) of about 5 percent and a reduction in triglycerides of about 10 percent. Like the LDL-cholesterol, triglycerides are a blood fat that when elevated, predicts the development of heart disease and stroke. Triglycerides tend to be high in people who do not exercise, are overweight, eat lots of sweets, and drink more than one alcoholic beverage per day, as well as in individuals with diabetes.

The alpha-adrenergic blockers can be added to other antihypertensive agents including diuretics, ACE inhibitors, and calcium channel blockers. It now appears (based on the data from ALLHAT) that alpha-blockers should be considered only when a second or third agent needs to be added to a blood pressure–lowering regime. Alpha-adrenergic blockers have been combined with beta-blockers to form a group of drugs called alpha–beta-blockers.

ALPHA-BETA RECEPTOR ANTAGONISTS

It makes sense to combine alpha and beta adrenergic receptor blockades for the treatment of high blood pressure. Only two drugs in this class are currently available: labetalol (Normodyne, Trandate) and carvedilol (Coreg). Because these two drugs are not exactly alike in terms of the extent to which each blocks the various alpha- and beta-adrenergic receptors, they tend to have differing side effects. Carvedilol (Coreg) is particularly interesting because in addition to its alpha and beta blocking properties, at high doses it also has some calcium channel blocking properties. The commonly used doses of these drugs are listed in Table 7.9.

Table 7.9 Alpha-Beta Receptor Antagonists (Blockers)

ALPHA-BETA RECEPTOR ANTAGONIST	USUAL TOTAL DAILY DOSAGE (MG/DAY)	NUMBER OF DOSES/DAY
Labetalol (Normodyne, Trandate)	100–1,200	2
Carvedilol (Coreg)	6.25–50	2

Labetalol and Aortic Dissection

Both of these drugs are good blood pressure–lowering medications. Labetalol is available in both an oral form and an intraveneous preparation. The intravenous form has been shown to be useful in the face of markedly elevated blood pressure and in the case of aortic dissection. Aortic dissection is a potentially deadly situation, which is most often the result of untreated (or inadequately treated) high blood pressure. In an aortic dissection, the inner layer of the aorta (the main artery carrying blood from the heart to all areas of the body) tears. As a result blood flows between the layers of the aorta and is unable to get out of the aorta to the body organs that need it. The blood from the heart, which is stuck between the walls or layers of the artery, actually puts pressure on the aorta and can cause it to collapse.

The symptoms a person experiences as a result of an aortic dissection depend entirely on where in the aorta the tear occurs. The most common symptoms include sudden onset of severe pain in the back (between the shoulder blades) or chest. Other people faint; still others develop very high blood pressure. In the worst situation a person can experience circulatory collapse and death.

Treatment of an aortic dissection is determined primarily by its location. Dissections occurring in the aorta as it exits the heart (ascending aorta) typically require emergency surgery, whereas those lower down are often treated with medications including labetalol. The awful thing about aortic dissection is that it is frequently fatal and it is totally preventable.

Just before I entered medical school, one of my favorite uncles collapsed and died of an aortic dissection. At the time I couldn't understand it. Uncle Ray was an incredibly vigorous man. He cut all his own wood. He hiked in the woods, he was lean, he and my Aunt Rita square danced every chance they could—sometimes five times a week. In short, he looked the picture of health. But much as I loved Uncle Ray, I have to admit he was a stubborn old Yankee who didn't believe in doctors, and he had probably had high blood pressure for most of his adult life. (They don't call it the silent killer for nothing.)

By the time Uncle Ray arrived at the hospital, there was little that could be done. He left my Aunt Rita just months before their fiftieth wedding anniversary. When I learned about aortic dissections during my third year of medical school, I wished I could turn back the hands of time. If you are putting off getting treatment for your high blood pressure, please see your doctor and take your medication. The people who love you will have you around a lot longer.

The oral form of labetalol has also been used to treat high blood pressure occurring during pregnancy. In general, however, labetalol has fallen out of favor primarily because of some of its unusual side effects, which include severe scalp itching and, in men, failure to ejaculate during intercourse. In addition, liver failure resulting in death has been very rarely reported. For this reason liver function tests (a blood test) should probably be done regularly by people on labetalol.

The intravenous form of labetalol has also been used in the treatment of a rare hormonal cause of high blood pressure called pheochromocytoma. Pheochromocytoma, which can cause wild fluctuations in blood pressure, is discussed in chapter 9.

Coreg and Heart Failure

Carvedilol (Coreg) is a newer alpha-beta adrenergic receptor blocker. There is little doubt that Coreg is capable of lowering blood pressure, as are all of the other agents we have discussed thus far. So why might your doctor choose Coreg over another agent? Coreg has been shown to be especially beneficial in people with congestive heart failure.

Who Should Take Them

As a group, elderly people do beautifully with the alpha–beta-receptor antagonists. Interestingly, when compared to a group of younger hypertensives, older people tend to require lower doses of these agents.

In addition, people with impaired kidney function should also be considered for the alpha–beta-receptor antagonists. This is primarily because the kidney does not metabolize this class of medications. Impaired kidney function, therefore, does not prevent their use. On the contrary, these drugs are almost totally metabolized by the liver, so they should be used with great caution by people with underlying liver disease. You might wonder if the issues described above regarding the alpha-blockers used in ALLHAT apply to Coreg. The answer appears to be no. Coreg is mostly a beta-blocker with a small amount of alpha blockade. It does not appear that this agent will increase the risk of cardiac events. In fact, it has been clearly shown to prevent cardiac events.

CENTRAL AND PERIPHERAL SYMPATHOLYTICS

This group of drugs blocks the effects of the sympathetic nervous system either at the level of the brain (central sympatholytics) or within the body (peripheral sympatholytics). An increase in sympathetic nervous system activity causes blood vessels to constrict and thus blood pressure rises. Blocking this sympathetic activity therefore leads to a significant reduction in blood pressure.

The currently available sympatholytics are listed in Table 7.10.

Central Sympatholytics: Side Effects and Use in Pregnancy

As a group, the central sympatholytics tend to have similar side effects. These side effects occur in up to 40 percent of people and are related to the fact that the drugs work within the brain. They include fatigue, sedation, and dry mouth. Although the side effect of fatigue and sedation would appear to be a negative one, it is sometimes useful, especially for people who have difficulty sleeping or for those who are very anxious, because these medications can have a calming effect. The dry mouth (caused by a reduction in saliva formation) can be very severe and at times can result in cavities and gum disease. (Your mouth is made to be moist.)

One problem with this group of drugs, with the exception of guanabenz (Wytensin), is that they cause fluid retention. As a result they are almost always given in association with a diuretic. In fact, in the 1960s through the 1970s diuretics and the central

Table 7.10 Central and Peripheral Sympatholytics

DRUG	USUAL TOTAL DAILY DOSAGE (MG/DAY)	NUMBER OF DOSES/DAY
Central Sympatholytics		
Clonidine (Catapres)[1]	0.2–0.6	2
Guanabenz (Wytensin)	8–32	2
Guanfacine (Tenex)[2]	1–3	1
Methyldopa (Aldomet)	500–3,000	2–4
Peripheral Sympatholytics		
Deserpidine (Harmonyl)[3]	0.25–0.5	1
Guanadrel (Hylorel)	10–75	2–3
Guanethidine (Ismelin)	10–50	1
Reserpine (Serpasil)	0.05–0.25	1

[1]Clonidine is also available in a transdermal patch form called Catapres TTS. The patch is applied to the skin once a week. The Catapres TTS system comes in three strengths: 2.5 mg, 5.0 mg, and 7.5 mg. The medication is absorbed slowly over the course of a week.
[2]Guanfacine (Tenex) is taken once daily at bedtime.
[3]Deserpidine (Harmonyl) is very rarely used.

sympatholytic, methyldopa (Aldomet), were the mainstay of blood pressure–lowering therapy.

Over time the central sympatholytics have fallen out of favor, and now they are infrequently used. The one exception is the transdermal preparation of clonidine (Catapres TTS), which has assumed a greater role, especially for older people.

In general methyldopa (Aldomet) is only used in the treatment of high blood pressure associated with pregnancy. Obviously there is a great reluctance to test new blood pressure medications in pregnant women, but methyldopa (Aldomet) has a long track record of "relative safety" in pregnancy and therefore continues to be used in this special situation. I find this a bit disturbing in some ways because methyldopa has been reported to cause a number of potentially life-threatening and unique side effects. These include fulminant liver disease and a severe form of anemia called Coombs-positive hemolytic anemia.

Finally, methyldopa can interfere with the effect of other medications including levodopa, bromocriptine, and monoamine oxidase inhibitors. (These drugs are rarely used in pregnancy, but are used in other situations. The monoamine oxidase inhibitors, in addition to being used to treat depression, are sometimes used to treat Parkinson's disease.) Unfortunately, when it comes to treating the relatively common situation of high blood pressure in pregnancy, it appears the philosophy is "better the devil you know." If one of the severe side effects occurs in a pregnant woman, it generally resolves when the drug is stopped.

I almost never prescribe oral clonidine (Catapres), but I frequently prescribe the transdermal (patch form) preparation of this drug. The patch is changed only once a week and provides a full week of coverage—no need to remember to take a pill. It is important to know that unlike the pill form, which lowers blood pressure within a half-hour, the patch may take a full day to take effect. Because the patch has a slower onset of action it also seems to have a milder side effect profile (less sedation, fatigue, and dry mouth). I suggest that the patch be placed on the chest or upper arm, as these locations appear to allow for the most even absorption.

One side effect unique to the patch is obviously skin irritation, which can occur in up to 20 percent of users. I generally recommend rotating the location of the patch from week to week (right arm, right chest, left chest, and left arm, then repeat). One of the most important and unique side effects of clonidine is rebound hypertension. This occurs to some extent with many blood pressure medications, but typically just involves a return of blood pressure to pretreatment levels. With clonidine the rebound may be severe, with blood pressure greatly exceeding pretreatment levels. This is especially the case if a person is also taking a beta-blocker.

On the other hand, clonidine has been used to treat many problems that may coexist in a person with high blood pressure. These include hot flashes due to menopause, withdrawal from morphine, diarrhea in diabetics (which is due to neuropathy of the intestinal tract), and restless leg syndrome. People with restless leg syndrome generally complain of inability to stop their legs from moving. Its cause is unknown; it can be very debilitating, and it is most troublesome at night.

Peripheral Sympatholytics

The peripheral sympatholytics block the transport of norepinephrine so less of this catecholamine is available to cause blood vessels to constrict. Remember, norepinephrine is a substance in the blood that when released from nerve endings has the ability to attach to receptors on blood vessels and make them constrict or clamp down, causing the blood pressure to rise.

Reserpine (Serpasil) became available in the 1940s and was the first peripheral sympatholytic introduced in the United States. It wasn't until the 1960s that this drug became quite popular. It was first derived from an Indian snakeroot, *Rauwolfia serpentina*. Reserpine has been reported to cause a number of side effects including depression, peptic ulcer disease, and nasal stuffiness, and it may exacerbate (cause to become active) ulcerative colitis. If reserpine (Serpasil) is used in low doses, the incidence of side effects is low. However, low doses of reserpine have only a modest impact on blood pressure. Often in order to minimize the side effects of reserpine, a tiny dose (0.05 mg per day) will be combined with a diuretic. The impact can be dramatic, often with full normalization of blood pressure.

Guanethidine (Ismelin) is another peripheral sympatholytic. In the past, before there were lots of once-a-day blood pressure medications, this drug was frequently used because of its long duration of action. It is not uncommon to find that increasing the dose of any blood pressure medication improves its ability to lower blood pressure. However, in almost all cases, at some point a higher dose causes additional side effects but no further blood pressure reduction. On the contrary, the greater the dose of guanethidine, the greater the reduction in blood pressure.

However, as with other agents, the side effects also increase. It is actually these attributes (which in the past were felt to be helpful) that are now the reason Ismelin is rarely used. Ismelin hangs around so long that if a person has an unwanted side effect it may take a prolonged time for it to go away. Certain drugs used in the treatment of depression (namely, tricyclic antidepressants such as nortriptyline) may prevent Ismelin from lowering blood pressure. Finally, in people taking monoamine oxidase inhibitors (either for depression or for the treatment of Parkinson's disease) the use of Ismelin can paradoxically cause severe high blood pressure. Other side effects include diarrhea and edema. People with edema will require the addition of a diuretic. And in men there is also the disturbing side effect of retrograde ejaculation (failure of semen to ejaculate during intercourse).

Guanadrel (Hylorel) is very similar to Ismelin except that it hangs around for a much shorter time. On the negative side, this means it must be taken two or three times a day. On the positive side, all of the side effects mentioned above are less pronounced.

Overall, as a class, the peripheral sympatholytics are infrequently used. Some people have speculated that the reason is that because they are generic and relatively inexpensive, drug companies are not pushing physicians to prescribe them. I don't think this is true; physicians still prescribe diuretics even though many are generic and cheap. I believe physicians are reluctant to prescribe the peripheral sympatholytics because of their potential side effects, when they have so many blood pressure agents with a low side effect profiles available. Although Ismelin is still used for the odd patient for whom nothing else has worked, in general these agents are not first-line blood pressure medications.

Direct Vasodilators

This group of drugs works by directly relaxing the walls of your blood vessels. The two direct vasodilators available in the United States include hydralazine (Apresoline) and minoxidil (Loniten).

The typical doses and number of doses required per day are listed in Table 7.11.

Table 7.11 Direct Vasodilators

DIRECT VASODILATOR	USUAL TOTAL DAILY DOSAGE (MG/DAY)	NUMBER OF DOSES/DAY
Hydralazine (Apresoline)	50–300	2
Minoxidil (Loniten)	5–100	1

General Side Effects

Because the direct vasodilators dilate the blood vessels of the skin (as well as elsewhere), it should be expected that as a group they might cause flushing (and indeed they do). Other common side effects of both hydralazine and minoxidil are fluid retention (both of these drugs should be taken in combination with a diuretic), headache, and palpitations. In addition to the side effects these two agents share, they also have effects that are unique.

Side Effects Unique to Hydralazine

Hydralazine is well known to cause a condition called "drug-induced lupus." This condition generally occurs after a person has been on hydralazine for at least six months. You have probably heard of lupus as a rheumatological disease that causes skin rash, joint pain, fatigue, weight loss, enlarged spleen, and kidney and heart problems. Both drug-induced lupus and lupus occurring in the absence of hydralazine are more common in women than men. Hydralazine-induced lupus seems to occur most often in people who metabolize this medication rather slowly. Fortunately the lupus seen in people on hydralazine quickly disappears when the drug is discontinued.

Conditions Unique to Minoxidil

Minoxidil is even more potent than hydralazine. Like hydralazine it is never given as a first-line medication and is almost always used as a fourth drug for a person with blood pressure that has failed to respond to three other medications. Because of the edema it causes in almost everyone, it should be given in combination with a diuretic. Minoxidil is used most commonly for people with advanced kidney disease in whom uncontrollable high blood pressure is a frequent problem.

Side Effects

Unlike hydralazine, minoxidil does not cause "drug-induced lupus." Minoxidil, however, has its own unique side effect that is loved by some and despised by others. It causes hypertrichosis, which is just another way of saying hair growth. This occurs especially on the face but also on the scalp. You can probably guess that the love/hate issue is evenly divided by sex. Men love it; women hate it. In fact, the hypertrichosis greatly limits the utility of this medication in women. Fortunately the hair growth is completely reversible, resolving within a few weeks of discontinuing the drug.

Minoxidil is also available as a very weak topical solution called Rogaine. Although Rogaine is unlikely to lower blood pressure, it can promote hair growth.

This complex chapter has reviewed the currently available classes of blood pressure–lowering medications and their mechanisms of action. The fact that so many different drug classes affect blood pressure speaks to the fact that blood pressure regulation is extremely complex and multifaceted.

It should not be surprising that the search for new classes of blood pressure–lowering agents continues. At this writing there are at least seven new classes of blood pressure–lowering medications (potassium channel openers, serotonin-related agents, dopamine agonists, renin inhibitors, imidazolines, neural endopeptidase inhibitors, and endothelin-receptor antagonists) at some stage of development. Some of these newer classes of medications are already available abroad. From my point of view this is great. Two people can have the same degree of blood pressure elevation, but for two very different reasons. Each needs a blood pressure medication that will treat the underlying cause of the blood pressure elevation. The greater the variety of medications available, the more likely it is that the appropriate drug for the appropriate person will be found.

In closing I would like to recap my general approach to the treatment of high blood pressure with medications. As previously mentioned, I hope that by the time I am considering the use of a blood pressure–lowering medication, my patient has already made many lifestyle changes including losing weight, developing an exercise program, limiting alcohol and salt, and increasing potassium-rich foods. If the problem is just high blood pressure and nothing else, the Joint National Committee on the Detection and Treatment of High Blood Pressure in Adults recommends that the initial medication choice be either a beta-blocker or a diuretic.

On the other hand, for people with various conditions other drugs should be chosen as first-line therapy. For example, in a person with a history of heart failure, I think ACE inhibitors, beta-blockers, or diuretics are wise choices. People who have previously suffered a heart attack should receive beta-blockers, ACE inhibitors, or a calcium channel blocker (either a dihydropyridine like amlodipine or the nondihydropyridine long-acting verapamil). People whose heart function has diminished following a heart attack clearly benefit from an ACE inhibitor. People with diabetes, especially those with protein in the urine, should be treated with an ACE inhibitor. It should be pointed out that diuretics and beta-blockers have been found to worsen blood sugar levels. Although both classes of drugs increase blood sugar levels, only beta-blockers have been implicated in increasing the risk of developing diabetes. In the elderly who may have only systolic hypertension (the systolic blood pressure [top number] is elevated while the diastolic pressure [bottom number] is normal) the best medications appear to be diuretics and dihydropyridine calcium channel blockers. For those people with high cholesterol levels, alpha-blockers actually improve cholesterol. (But based on ALLHAT, the alpha-blockers should not be used as a first-line blood pressure–lowering medication.) ACE inhibitors and calcium channel blockers are lipid (cholesterol) neutral. On the other hand, diuretics and beta-blockers worsen cholesterol levels.

People with palpitations, anxiety, hyperthyroidism, hand tremor, and migraine headaches have all been found to benefit from beta-blockers. (In this situation the beta-blocker helps the underlying problem and improves their blood pressure as well.) A man with an enlarged prostate may lower his blood pressure and shrink his prostate with the use of an alpha-blocker. Finally, a woman with osteoporosis (thinning of the bones) may protect her bones as she lowers her blood pressure with a diuretic.

As you endeavor to normalize your blood pressure, it is crucial for you to work closely with your doctor. Request that low doses of a blood pressure medication be used initially and be willing to gradually increase the dose of the chosen medication. At some point your doctor may need to change the medication because it isn't working or to add a second or even a third medication. The goal should be perfect blood pressure control with the fewest possible side effects. As I mentioned earlier, in the interest of good control, it may be necessary to put up with some minor side effects, but this should be the exception rather than the rule. If you keep at it, there is little doubt that you will be able to dramatically improve your blood pressure, which will in turn dramatically reduce your risk of heart disease and stroke.

CHAPTER 8

HOME BLOOD PRESSURE MONITORS

So you have high blood pressure and you want to follow your progress as you implement changes in your diet, salt intake, and exercise and alcohol consumption. Or perhaps your doctor has already put you on a blood pressure medication and you want to see how well it is working. Or it could be that your doctor suspects "white coat hypertension" and wants to see what your blood pressure runs at home.

For any one of these reasons, you make up your mind to purchase a home blood pressure monitor. This seems like a sensible and simple idea, so you head to the store and are confronted with dozens of models to choose from. How can you possibly know which one to buy?

You can't. Blood pressure can fluctuate significantly in a given person over the course of the day. And so, since you have just made some changes aimed at lowering your pressure, you can't even try out the cuffs and say, "This one is closest to my true reading." You don't know what your true reading is at the moment. In any case, there is little doubt that your trip to the store has already raised your blood pressure!

EVALUATING HOME MONITOR CUFFS

When my patients ask me which blood pressure cuff they should purchase I explain that since there are many good cuffs available, the important thing is finding the one that is right for them. For example, a mechanical blood pressure cuff is an economical and excellent choice for many. But good hearing and manual dexterity (you must be able to put on a blood pressure cuff, pump it full of air, then listen with a stethoscope) are a must in order to use this type of monitor accurately. The manual monitors generally cost between $25 and $30.

For people who have trouble hearing or who find the mechanical cuff awkward to work with, the electronic blood pressure monitors are an excellent alternative. There are three different types: those that fit on the arm just above the elbow, on the wrist, and on the finger. Overall, the further away you move from the heart, the less accurate the cuffs become. In other words, the arm models are the most consistent and accurate; the finger models are the least likely to give you a true reading. The wrist models are somewhere in between. I do not advise purchasing a finger model, which incidentally are the most expensive. The arm models cost anywhere from about $50 to $100 and the wrist models generally between $110 and $135.

If you purchase an electronic blood pressure cuff, make sure to find out if you can return it if it is found to be inaccurate. How can you tell? Bring your cuff to your doctor's office and ask to have the cuff checked against your doctor's manual cuff. If you know your blood pressure is the same in both arms, your pressure can be taken simultaneously in both arms—one side with your new monitor and the other using your doctor's mercury device. Alternatively, as long as you rest for at least 15 seconds between measurements you can measure your blood pressure sequentially. This way of evaluating your cuff may be a little less accurate, but it is still acceptable; blood pressure should be very similar for both readings. If anything, you should expect the second reading to be slightly lower than the first. If the results from the two cuffs are relatively close, you can feel confident about bringing the cuff home.

As you know from reading the earlier chapters of this book, blood pressure is recorded as systolic over diastolic pressure. The systolic pressure reflects the pressure in your arteries as the heart is squeezing blood out. The diastolic pressure is a measure of the pressure within the artery between beats, when the heart is relaxing.

If you are using a manual cuff, you pump air into the cuff to the point at which you can no longer feel your pulse. Listen with a stethoscope over the artery at the bend in your arm. When you hear the first sound, look at the gauge attached to the cuff. The number you see at that moment is your systolic blood pressure. Continue to let air out of the cuff until you no longer hear your pulse. The number on the gauge at this point is your diastolic blood pressure.

The electronic cuffs are easier. In general, you slip the cuff on your arm or wrist. The cuff inflates either manually or electronically. Air is then slowly released from the cuff. Once the cuff is fully deflated you will see an easy to read digital display of both your systolic and diastolic blood pressure.

Consumer Reports (October, 1996) published a well-conducted review of currently available blood pressure cuffs. The report reviews five manual monitors, eleven electronic arm models, four electronic wrist models, and two electronic finger models.

All the manual models were found to be excellent. (But remember, these are only as accurate as your own ears.) The manual models included the Omron HEM–18, the Lumiscope 100-021, the Walgreens 2001, the Marshall 104, and the Sunmark 100.

The best electronic arm models were the AND UA-702 and the Omron HEM-712C. Both of these models were given the

Consumer Reports "Best Buy" rating. Although none of the wrist models achieved "Best Buy" status, the two best were the Omron HEM-605 and the Omron HEM-601. All of these models are currently on the market. You can obtain a copy of the report by calling *Consumer Reports* at 1-800-234-1645. Your local library may also have the report (probably in the microfilm collection).

As you measure your blood pressure at home or at work it is important to remember that your blood pressure can be quite volatile. Many things you do can have a predictable impact on blood pressure. In a study of 461 people with high blood pressure (not treated with medications) Clark and colleagues found that sleep dramatically reduces blood pressure. On the other hand, meetings and work result in a significant increase in blood pressure. As compared to relaxing while awake, sleeping was found to reduce the systolic and diastolic blood pressures by 10 and 7.6 mmHg, respectively. Again as compared to relaxing, meetings resulted in a 20.0/15.0 mmHg rise in systolic and diastolic blood pressure. Work was not much better, leading to an increase of 16.0/13.0 mmHg in the systolic and diastolic pressures. Other activities resulting in substantial increases in both systolic and diastolic blood pressures include driving, walking, dressing, doing chores, and talking on the phone. I guess the moral of the story is we should all stay home in our pajamas all day.

Since there is little chance that you can or want to remain idle all day, it is crucial to work on lifestyle changes and take blood pressure medications when necessary. You cannot prevent your blood pressure from fluctuating with various activities, but your goal should be fluctuation within the normal range.

As you begin to measure your blood pressure at home or at work it is important to develop a good technique. Using either the mechanical or electronic cuff, make sure you are sitting upright with your back supported (in a chair with a back). Your arm should also be supported (your forearm on a table or desk). The cuff around your upper arm should be level with your heart. It is best if you wear a short-sleeve shirt, but a thin long-sleeve shirt is acceptable. Don't wear thick or tight tops when measuring your blood pressure. Measure your arm circumference; if it is greater than 33 cm (13.2 inches), you will need to purchase a large cuff. An incorrect cuff size can lead to an overestimation of the blood pressure.

If you have opted to monitor your blood pressure with a manual cuff it is important to deflate the cuff correctly (at a rate of 2 to 4 mmHg per second). Deflating more slowly may cause erroneously high readings. It is also crucial to measure your blood pressure in a quiet room. Noise won't interfere with accuracy when you are using an electronic device, but it can be a major factor when you are trying to measure your own pressure using a stethoscope.

No matter what type of cuff you are using, remember—immediately following a caffeinated or alcoholic beverage, blood pressure rises. Blood pressure also increases in response to cigarette smoking.

In certain situations your doctor may suggest using ambulatory blood pressure monitoring (ABPM). If your doctor prescribes ABPM, you will wear a standard blood pressure cuff that is attached to a small pump. This cuff is automatically inflated every fifteen minutes during the day and every thirty minutes at night. The blood pressures are stored in memory for later evaluation. I sometimes use ABPM when a person does not seem to be responding adequately to the blood pressure medications I have prescribed. In this situation I need to determine if the person really has responded but gets nervous in my office. I also use ABPM when a person has perfectly controlled blood pressure in my office but complains of dizziness and fatigue at home. In this situation, do I have this person on too much medication? If I suspect that a person has an underlying disorder that results in periodic high blood pressure, ABPM is useful. ABPM is also helpful in making the diagnosis of "white coat hypertension." If I see a person with very high blood pressure in my office but no evidence of problems related to high blood pressure (that is, no kidney- or heart-related problems), I may wonder what her blood pressure is like throughout the day. In some cases it turns out that she has totally normal blood pressure everywhere but in my office. This person doesn't need medications.

Leo is one of my favorite patients. I met him about eight years ago when I was asked to see him for cardiac risk factor reduction following his bypass surgery. At that time, he was overweight and sedentary. His diet was poor and he had high blood pressure, borderline diabetes, and high cholesterol. Thankfully he had quit smoking many years earlier. I always start by trying to determine how motivated a person is to make changes. From the minute I met Leo I knew he was motivated. His wife had died a number of years ago. He lived with his daughter whom he obviously adored, and he told me that since he didn't want his daughter to be an orphan (she was forty-two at the time), he would do anything I asked.

We talked about the need for him to develop a regular exercise program. I suggested he begin with the Cardiac Rehabilitation Program at the New England Heart Institute. I explained that the rehabilitation program would give him the confidence he needed to develop a lifelong exercise program. In his case cardiac rehabilitation would last twelve weeks, and he would exercise in a structured environment. This would allow him to work with the nurses and exercise physiologists as he decided what his exercise routine would be upon graduation from cardiac rehabilitation. Anyone who participates in cardiac rehabilitation at the New England Heart Institute is given an exercise prescription for life. This allows people to work toward achieving a safe target heart rate and level of energy expenditure.

Next we talked about his diet. I recommended a salt-restricted, low-fat, low-sugar, calorie-restricted diet. (See chapter 3.) We specifically talked about the importance of avoiding some of the very salty, high-fat foods (bacon, potato chips, salad dressings) that Leo consumed on a daily basis.

Because of his underlying heart disease I started Leo on a beta-blocker to control his high blood pressure, which was running about 160/90 mmHg while he was in the hospital. I told him that ultimately he might require a medication for his cholesterol and another for his blood sugar. We would decide this over the next few months.

Leo was as good as his word. Over the next three months he lost 20 pounds (which he has kept off to this day). His diet improved dramatically. The cardiac rehabilitation staff loved him. Upon graduation from cardiac rehabilitation he began walking three miles in the morning and another three in mid-afternoon. (Again, he continues to this day.) His cholesterol level and his blood sugar were perfect. But his blood pressure was 200/110 mmHg. I repeated the blood pressure measurement several times; it never dropped below 190/100 mmHg. Leo told me that on his home cuff his blood pressure was routinely 130–140/76–82 mmHg. Of course I asked him if his cuff had ever been tested against a cuff in a doctor's office. It hadn't. I called the staff at cardiac rehabilitation to ask if Leo had ever had blood pressure readings similar to the ones I was getting. They told me that on his first day of cardiac rehabilitation he had been high at 166/90 mmHg, but that his readings had been great for the subsequent twelve weeks. While this gave me some reassurance, I didn't feel right sending him out into the world with a blood pressure of 200/110 mmHg. I doubled his beta-blocker dose and asked him to go home and bring back his home cuff for evaluation. When he returned his home cuff read 190/100, as did our cuff. We now knew his cuff was accurate and getting very different readings in our office than in his home. (Again, this was reassuring.) He told me that as he left our office he could feel his blood pressure drop. When he was in our office, he explained, he was "so nervous." He said the more he tried to relax, the more nervous he became. His pulse in our office was 100/minute.

Over the next two weeks Leo called a number of times to tell me that he felt washed out and dizzy. His home blood pressure was reading 100/60 mmHg. I decided that maybe doubling the dose of his beta-blocker was not the right thing to do. I asked him to come in and be hooked up to a twenty-four-hour ABPM. He agreed. On the increased dose of the beta-blocker his blood pressure was indeed exceedingly low, sometimes dipping to 90/60 mmHg. And he was symptomatic with the dips, complaining of dizziness and fatigue. As an experiment we had him come into our office, go grocery shopping, go to the bank, walk his three miles, and drive in traffic while wearing the ABPM device. The only time his blood pressure soared was in my office. Case closed.

We reduced his blood pressure medication back to his old dose. I do not check his blood pressure anymore—he brings in his home readings and we use these. Twice a year we have him bring his home machine in to be calibrated against ours, but it is done on my day off. Leo and I have a great relationship, yet he cannot explain why he gets so nervous when he comes to see me. He has, however, noticed that now that our visits involve only an evaluation of his heart and a check of his cholesterol and blood sugar, he is much more relaxed. If I had only Leo's office readings to go on I can only guess how many medications he would be on, and how awful he might feel.

If you have found a huge discrepancy between your home and doctor's office blood pressure readings, ABPM might be useful. Unfortunately ABPM has not taken off in the United States for the simple reason that most insurance companies refuse to pay for it. While I don't think it should be used indiscriminately, it can be a very important tool in cases like Leo's.

PART III

MANAGING BLOOD PRESSURE IN SPECIAL SITUATIONS

CHAPTER 9

🙠

WHEN NOTHING SEEMS TO WORK

High blood pressure that does not respond to conventional treatments is often called "refractory hypertension." Refractory hypertension is generally defined as a blood pressure above 140/90mmHg despite adequate doses of three blood pressure medications (one of which should be a diuretic). For people with diabetes and kidney disease, blood pressure is considered refractory at 130/85 mmHg. An isolated elevation of the systolic blood pressure above 160mmHg despite three medications should be considered refractory hypertension in an elderly person. As you may recall, many elderly men and women have elevations only of the systolic blood pressure.

Before considering diseases of the kidney, blood vessels, adrenal, thyroid, and parathyroid glands, disorders such as sleep apnea, and conditions such as severe obesity (which can cause severe refractory high blood pressure), it is important to mention some of the most common causes of difficult-to-control high blood pressure that may mimic true refractory hypertension.

Before you accept that you have refractory hypertension, make sure that whoever is checking your blood pressure is using the appropriate size blood pressure cuff. If a person's arm measures greater than 33 centimeters (13.2 inches) in circumference at a point approximately two to three inches above the elbow, a large blood pressure cuff must be used, because a standard size cuff can significantly overestimate the blood pressure. In such a situation refractory hypertension might be incorrectly diagnosed.

Sometimes refractory blood pressure will be diagnosed when blood pressure is repeatedly measured immediately after drinking a caffeinated beverage or after smoking a cigarette. A general rule is to wait thirty minutes after caffeine or nicotine before assessing blood pressure. Of course, I believe it is my duty to point out that quitting smoking altogether, rather than just waiting for thirty minutes, is a better solution! Remember, if your blood pressure rises dramatically after a cigarette and you smoke twenty to thirty cigarettes per day, your blood pressure may be elevated most of the time.

And sometimes a person just needs a little time (usually five minutes) to relax in a quiet room before the blood pressure is measured. In a busy clinic or doctor's office, this simple measure is occasionally overlooked.

In addition to the causes noted above, some elderly people have such stiff arteries that the blood pressure cuff fails to work properly. Many times they are thought to have refractory hypertension in spite of having all the symptoms of marked hypotension (low blood pressure), such as dizziness, confusion and even chest pain. For these people we sometimes have to insert a catheter directly into an artery to get a true blood pressure reading. Many of them will have their medications either discontinued or dramatically decreased. They will feel better, too.

What about "white coat hypertension"? Some people have perfectly controlled blood pressure everywhere but the doctor's office. People with "white coat hypertension" may be more likely to develop true high blood pressure than someone who is always found to have a normal blood pressure reading. However, a person in this situation does not have true refractory hypertension. A good way to determine if a person really only has high blood pressure readings at the doctor's office (as opposed to high blood pressure in response to any stressful situation) is to evaluate blood pressure with an ambulatory monitor.

Before looking for rare diseases that might be responsible for the refractory blood pressure, your doctor will want to know if you are using any prescription or nonprescription drugs that might increase your blood pressure. These drugs, including birth control pills, steroids, decongestants, many diet pills (especially those containing phenylpropanolamine), cyclosporin, nonsteroidal anti-inflammatory medications, and gold therapy, were reviewed in chapter 2. In addition, cocaine and amphetamines can cause marked increases in blood pressure. If blood pressure is assessed soon after exposure to these drugs, it can seem to be refractory.

In some cases excessive dietary intake of salt may make it impossible for blood pressure medications to normalize your pressure. I have had patients on three blood pressure–lowering medications who were able to come off one or two when they reduced their salt intake. Alcohol (in excess of two to three drinks per day) can make it impossible to control blood pressure. Finally, licorice/salt candies can wreak havoc with blood pressure control. These tend to be consumed primarily in Europe but if you eat this type of candy, be aware of the potential consequences.

Last but certainly not least, before refractory hypertension can be diagnosed it is important to be honest with yourself regarding how often you miss your medications. If it is a frequent occurrence, speak frankly to your doctor. Do you miss them because their timing makes them hard to remember? If so, your doctor may be able to devise an easier dosing schedule or have you switch to a once-a-day medication.

Or do you skip doses because the expense of the drug is too high? If this is the case, don't be embarrassed. Speak openly to your doctor. Ask about generic drugs or patient assistance programs. Living on a fixed income or having no insurance can make it very difficult to afford costly medications. You will be much better off being open with your doctor. In fact, being honest will save you from the unnecessary additional expense of tests to figure out why your blood pressure is so resistant to the medications your doctor thinks you are taking!

Finally, sometimes doctors fail to give a dose that is high enough to be effective. Although I am in favor of starting any medication at the lowest possible dose, if a drug is working but hasn't gotten you down to the numbers you require, it should be increased to the maximum dose unless you experience intolerable side effects.

If none of the above applies to you, if you are taking three blood pressure–lowering medications at the maximum or near maximum dose and your blood pressure is still higher than the levels described above, it is crucial that you be evaluated for the presence of secondary causes of high blood pressure.

RENAL HYPERTENSION

The most common cause of "secondary hypertension" is underlying kidney disease. In fact, most significant kidney disease is ultimately complicated by hypertension. Sometimes it is difficult to determine which came first: the kidney disease or the high blood pressure. There is no doubt that kidney disease, no matter what the cause, leads to high blood pressure. Conversely, high blood pressure may also cause kidney damage. Once the kidneys have been damaged by the high blood pressure, it may actually be the kidney disease that causes a worsening of blood pressure control!

But no matter what the underlying cause of the kidney disease, careful control of blood pressure can slow further kidney damage and reduce the risk of developing heart disease. Since most people with end-stage kidney disease ultimately die of heart disease, blood pressure control is crucial.

Although there are many diseases that adversely affect kidney function, there are only so many ways that the kidney damage can cause high blood pressure. In general, a damaged kidney is less able to rid the body of excess sodium. Sodium and fluids are retained and high blood pressure develops as a result of volume overload. Over time, chronic volume overload can lead to an increase in the stiffness of a person's arteries. This stiffness (or resistance) makes it harder for blood to flow freely in the arteries, and high blood pressure is perpetuated and can become worse. Finally, people with kidney disease may experience reduced ability to inactivate circulating blood pressure–raising hormones. This again contributes to high blood pressure.

It also appears that people with underlying kidney disease may not experience a drop in blood pressure during sleep. As a rule such a drop is natural for all of us. A loss of this diurnal drop in blood pressure exposes the body to higher blood pressure around the clock and may contribute to further kidney damage.

Multiple different disorders can lead to chronic kidney disease. These include common causes such as diabetes and chronic infection, as well as somewhat less common conditions such as polycystic kidney disease, glomerulonephritis, and drug-induced renal disease. Finally, occasionally a rare kidney tumor may secrete renin, which as you now know can lead to the constriction of a person's blood vessels and high blood pressure.

At times, as I have said, it is difficult to tell which came first, the high blood pressure or the kidney disease. Fortunately, if blood pressure–lowering medications are used early, it is often possible to prevent the worsening of both kidney function and blood pressure. This is especially true in the case of diabetic kidney disease.

Unfortunately many people may have very extensive kidney disease and markedly elevated blood pressure before they come to medical attention. These are the people who might be on three or four blood pressure medications and still have high blood pressure. In such a situation it may be necessary to institute dialysis (which will often itself improve blood pressure) and await a kidney transplant.

In a person with underlying kidney disease leading to hypertension it may be virtually impossible to improve blood pressure without sodium restriction. A high-salt diet can dramatically blunt the impact of most blood pressure–lowering medications, with the exception of the calcium channel blockers. In addition to salt restriction, people with chronic kidney disease and high blood pressure should restrict protein. Protein restriction tends to slow the progression of kidney disease and ultimately prevent a worsening of blood pressure.

If a person with severe kidney disease, who is on three or four blood pressure medications, still has high blood pressure, it is important to make sure that the right medications are being used and that the effectiveness of these medications is not being thwarted by poor dietary choices (i.e., a high-protein, high-sodium diet).

In general, the treatment of blood pressure in people with underlying kidney disease begins with sodium restriction. Diuretics are added, but it is important to note that if a person's creatinine level (a blood test that reflects kidney function) is above 2.5 mg/dl, thiazide diuretics are likely to be ineffective. (See chapter 7.) When diuretics are used, one of the so-called loop diuretics such as furosemide (Lasix) or torsemide (Demadex) would be a good choice. Both Lasix and Demadex need to be taken at least twice a day. Metolazone (Zaroxolyn) is a diuretic powerful enough to be used in the face of advanced kidney disease. ACE inhibitors are routinely used to treat high blood pressure in people with underlying kidney disease. Since most ACE inhibitors (with the exception of fosinopril [Monopril] which is excreted by the liver) are excreted by the kidney, their dose should be decreased in people with significant kidney disease. The ACE inhibitors have been shown to reduce protein loss by the kidneys. Likewise, calcium channel blockers are highly effective. In general there is no need to reduce the dose of a calcium channel blocker in the face of kidney disease.

If a person with underlying kidney disease fails to correct his blood pressure with the aforementioned dietary changes, a diuretic, an ACE inhibitor, and a calcium channel blocker, then perhaps minoxidil (Loniten) should be added. If minoxidil is used, generally both a loop diuretic and beta-blocker are also added to prevent the side effects of edema and rapid heart rate, respectively.

Very rarely, a single nonfunctioning kidney is the source of refractory high blood pressure. In such a case, it may be impossible to correct blood pressure without surgical removal of the diseased kidney. This approach is more likely to be effective in renovascular hypertension (see next section) than in hypertension due to the kidneys themselves.

Polycystic kidney disease is an inherited condition that can lead to multiple cysts in the kidneys and is a common cause of end-stage renal disease. Not surprisingly, polycystic kidney disease can cause very difficult-to-treat high blood pressure. It is important to make the diagnosis of this condition, because in addition to medications to control blood pressure, it is clear that either aspiration (drainage) or surgical excision of the cysts can frequently make a positive difference.

Diabetes is probably the most common cause of severe kidney disease in the United States. The first step in therapy is improvement in blood sugar level. Improved diabetes control will slow the loss of kidney function, which in turn will make blood pressure easier to control. But it must be said that blood pressure control in the diabetic can be extraordinarily difficult. After exhausting the previously outlined blood pressure medications and dietary changes, many diabetics do end up on chronic dialysis. This often results in an improvement in blood pressure, but ultimately many of these patients will require a kidney transplant.

Transplant recipients may develop severe high blood pressure from the surgery itself. Sometimes the kidney artery develops scarring where the transplanted kidney is sewn to the existing artery. In such a case, further surgery may be necessary. Sometimes the medications required to prevent rejection of the kidney themselves cause high blood pressure. Finally, if the kidney donor had high blood pressure, the recipient is more likely to develop posttransplant hypertension. In these latter two situations medications may substantially lower blood pressure.

In summary, "refractory hypertension" as a result of kidney disease may require multiple medications and at times may even require dialysis, transplantation, and in very rare cases, the removal of a single diseased kidney.

RENOVASCULAR HYPERTENSION

Although renovascular (blockages of the kidney arteries) hypertension is itself very uncommon, it is one of the most common causes of secondary hypertension. Blood pressure can rise dramatically in the face of a partial or complete blockage of the main renal (kidney) artery. High blood pressure can occur when one or both kidney arteries are affected.

If the artery to one kidney is blocked and the other is normal, the elevation in blood pressure is the result of an increase in renin production by the affected kidney. Remember, elevations in blood levels of renin lead to elevations in angiotensin II levels. Angiotensin II has a powerful constricting effect on blood vessels. When blood vessels constrict or clamp down, blood pressure rises. On the other hand, when the main artery to both kidneys is blocked the blood pressure elevation is in part related to increased renin levels, but even more to the inability of either kidney to get rid of sodium and fluids. People in this situation are at risk not only of severe high blood pressure and kidney failure, but also of fluid buildup in the lungs, a life-threatening crisis.

It is important to say at the outset that not everyone with a blockage in one or both of the kidney arteries will have renovascular hypertension. In fact, in the general population of people without high blood pressure, some studies have found as many as 32 percent have some narrowing of their renal arteries. In a group of people with high blood pressure, as many as 60 percent can be expected to have narrowing of the blood vessels. For most people the narrowing does not result in uncontrollable high blood pressure or have a major adverse impact on kidney function.

If a person with significant blockage in one or both renal arteries nonetheless has easy-to-control blood pressure and normal kidney function, then the only treatment required is to continue monitoring both blood pressure and kidney function. On the other hand, blockage of one or both of the main renal arteries can cause a rapid deterioration in kidney function and refractory hypertension. In such a case, more heroic therapies (which we will review shortly) should be considered.

You might be wondering how the kidney arteries become blocked in the first place. There are many causes, and a person's age and clinical history are good predictors of which is the most likely.

By far the most common cause of blockages in the arteries of the kidneys is cholesterol deposits. Cholesterol, as you know, can also block arteries of the heart, the legs, and the carotid arteries (leading to the brain). Frequently patients with cholesterol deposits in their kidney arteries are over the age of fifty, have elevated cholesterol, smoke, have diabetes, and have long-standing high blood pressure that has suddenly (as the blockage became severe) become difficult to control.

Other causes of renovascular hypertension include fibromuscular dysplasia and external compression of the renal artery or arteries. Fibromuscular dysplasia is a disorder that typically affects young women. For some unknown reason one of the three layers of the kidney artery or arteries enlarges and blocks blood flow in the affected artery. Women with fibromuscular dysplasia typically develop very high, very resistant blood pressure over a short period of time. In general the treatment for these women involves surgery or angioplasty (see below), because these procedures can be curative. Finally, blood flow to a single kidney artery (or both) can be blocked by external compression from, for example, a tumor. In such a case, therapy is directed toward the tumor or whatever is causing the compression.

As I have already mentioned, there are really two forms of renovascular hypertension: unilateral and bilateral (meaning the involvement of one or both kidneys). In general people with unilateral renovascular hypertension (one kidney involved) can be treated with a medicine (such as an ACE inhibitor) that blocks the impact of angiotensin II. In this situation, the ACE inhibitor's action of lowering the blood pressure also protects the normal kidney from damage. Calcium channel blockers are also useful in treating unilateral renovascular hypertension.

It is important that the medications be used in doses sufficient to normalize blood pressure. In some cases one or more medications will be required. If you have renovascular hypertension controlled with medications, your kidney function should be closely monitored (with blood tests). If kidney function begins to deteriorate or your blood pressure becomes very difficult to control with medicine, your doctor might want to consider opening your kidney artery with either surgery or angioplasty. (These procedures are discussed more fully below.)

Many people in whom blood flow to both kidneys is compromised (bilateral renovascular hypertension) will also do well with medications, as the arteries may not be completely blocked. The ACE inhibitors may lower the blood pressure beautifully for such patients. However, in the case of bilateral renal artery stenosis, ACE inhibitors may cause an abrupt reduction in kidney function. ACE inhibitors lower blood pressure by dilating blood vessels; this in turn reduces blood flow within the vessel. If there is a large blockage in an artery, that artery will no longer dilate but will experience a reduction in blood flow. True, the blood pressure declines, but the affected kidney does not receive enough blood flow, and its ability to function declines dramatically. In this situation, alternative blood pressure medications might be chosen or your doctor may want to consider surgery or angioplasty.

Although no study can absolutely determine if a person will benefit from angioplasty or surgery, some tests can help and are important to do. The test that is generally done first is a kidney ultrasound. This is a painless test that uses sound waves to determine the size of the kidneys. In the case of unilateral renovascular hypertension, the typical finding is a significantly smaller kidney on the side with the diseased renal artery. In bilateral renovascular disease both kidneys may be reduced in size.

If an abnormality is found on the ultrasound, the next step is generally a "captopril augmented renal scan." A simple renal scan can evaluate blood flow to the kidneys. The captopril augmented renal scan takes advantage of the fact that a single dose of captopril (which is an ACE inhibitor) can cause a marked temporary deterioration in kidney function on the side with the blockage. A person's response to the captopril augmented renal scan helps determine if she will be likely to benefit from surgery or angioplasty.

Some centers are now using either computed tomography (CT) or magnetic resonance imaging (MRI) studies to evaluate kidney function.

If your doctor is convinced that you have renovascular hypertension and is fairly certain you should be treated with either an angioplasty or surgery, he is likely to order an arteriogram as the initial study following the ultrasound. An arteriogram involves injecting a dye into the renal arteries. A blockage is obvious because the dye fails to pass through the site of the blockage. It is important to point out that because a blockage, even when present, is not always the cause of the high blood pressure, surgery to bypass it or angioplasty to open it up might not cure the blood pressure.

In the end, your doctor will probably use some of the tests described above in conjunction with your personal history (for example, did your high blood pressure suddenly develop or suddenly become impossible to control?) to help determine if surgery, angioplasty, or medication is the best way to treat your renovascular hypertension.

Traditionally surgery and/or angioplasty have been reserved for use in people with blood pressure nonresponsive to multiple medications in adequate doses, or who simply have dreadful side effects from medications. In some cases surgery or angioplasty is recommended to prevent the kidneys from losing function. And in some rare cases, interventions such as surgery and angioplasty are useful to treat people who refuse to take their medications as directed.

As mentioned earlier, the captopril augmented renal scan is useful in determining if someone is a good candidate for surgery or angioplasty. In general, young women with fibromuscular dysplasia have a great response to either procedure. People who have only a single blockage in their renal artery, especially if it is located in the middle, do much better with angioplasy or surgery than do people with multiple blockages.

If you require renal artery bypass surgery your doctor will need to decide how to perform the surgery. In some cases a vein from the leg (saphenous vein) or an artery from below the stomach will be used to connect the aorta to a point just beyond the renal artery blockage. In some cases none of the patient's own arteries are usable, and so a synthetic graft is used to connect the aorta to the renal artery. Some people may have severe blockages in the aorta too. In such cases, the bypass may connect a spleen or liver artery to the kidney artery. If angioplasty is to be used to open the artery, a hollow tube called a catheter with a balloon on its tip is threaded into the renal artery. When it reaches the blockage, the balloon is inflated and the blockage is broken up. Sometimes a metal spring called a stent is left at the site of the blockage to help prevent its recurrence.

The idea that surgery or angioplasty might cure renovascular hypertension makes these procedures very tempting. For some time they were widely recommended and performed without any studies comparing their outcome with that of medical (drug) therapy. Many people were also convinced that surgery was a safer and more definitive procedure than angioplasty. It is possible that this was true in the past, but with the advent of stents (metal springs that keep an artery open following angioplasty), the two procedures are likely roughly comparable.

Neither angioplasty nor surgery is risk free. A certain percentage of people actually get worse following these procedures. In general this is because of the unavoidable risk associated with these therapies. Sometimes the dye used to diagnose the renal artery blockages will worsen kidney function. At other times the surgery or angioplasty simply dislodges the cholesterol deposits from one artery, only to have them block smaller arteries somewhere else.

The soon-to-be-published DRASTIC Study compared treatment of renal artery stenosis patients with either angioplasty or medical therapy (medications). The results showed no clear benefit in favor of angioplasty with regard to either blood pressure or kidney function. This is not always the case, of course. You may have a form of renal artery stenosis that will respond beautifully to surgery or angioplasty.

And in some cases the likely benefits of surgery or angioplasty outweigh the potential risks associated with the procedure. Here is an example of a woman who had a great deal to gain from her angioplasty.

June is a sixty-four-year-old woman who was referred to my group because her doctor (who happened to be my husband, Tom) had diagnosed new and very difficult-to-control high blood pressure. Tom and I had discussed her case at home. By the time I met

June, I was convinced that she would probably benefit from a renal artery angioplasty.

Tom's notes explained that until six months earlier, June's blood pressure had been 130/70 mmHg. He also mentioned that for an unrelated reason, she had undergone a CT scan of her abdomen two years earlier. The kidneys in that scan were both reported as normal. As part of her current evaluation, Tom had ordered another kidney ultrasound. Unlike the earlier scan, the new one revealed that her right kidney was now considerably smaller than her left.

Tom also pointed out to me that her creatinine level had gotten markedly worse over the last six months and that her physical exam had changed. When he listened to her abdomen he noted a "bruit," a whooshing sound that occurs when blood traveling in an artery encounters a partial blockage. As the blood tries to pass, the flow becomes turbulent and creates extra noise or sound.

Tom had left very little for me to do. I ordered an angiogram and, just as we suspected, the study revealed blockages in both renal arteries. We suspected that both arteries were involved because of the fact that her kidney function had been deteriorating over the past few months. Generally, blood tests of kidney function are not adversely affected unless both arteries are a problem. June underwent bilateral (both sides) renal artery angioplasties with a stent in each artery. The results were excellent and she recovered beautifully. Unfortunately, she wasn't able to discontinue all her blood pressure medications, but she is now only on one medication (2 mg per day of Mavik, an ACE inhibitor) instead of three.

On the other hand, some people are at very high risk of a bad outcome with either surgery or angioplasty. In such a situation many specialists hold off doing any procedure until the benefits clearly outweigh the risks. Martin is a patient of mine who has bilateral renal artery blockages. I have been following him closely for the last four years. Six years ago, at the age of seventy-six, he underwent bypass surgery. He did well after the surgery but took a long time to recover and was not anxious, in his words, "to go under the knife again."

At the time of his bypass surgery he was noted to have a complete blockage of his left renal artery. Nothing was done about it because his blood pressure was fairly well controlled (140/82 mmHg) on two medications and his renal function was normal. Two years after his bypass surgery he was noted to have a rising creatinine level. His doctor suspected that this indicated that his right renal artery was now blocked. An angiogram proved this suspicion to be absolutely correct.

In addition, he was now on high doses of four blood pressure medications to maintain a blood pressure of 150/80 mgHG. His doctor suggested that Martin consider either surgery or angioplasty of his right renal artery. He was not suggesting it to help improve the blood pressure, but rather to prevent Martin's kidney function from deteriorating further. In general, when someone with a longstanding blockage in one artery develops a blockage in the other renal artery, the most you can hope for with a procedure is to prevent further kidney damage. It is highly unlikely that blood pressure will dramatically improve.

Martin, however, had other thoughts. He decided he would not undergo either surgery or an angioplasty. He reasoned that he was now seventy-eight with many health problems. He was a former smoker with chronic lung problems, he had prostate cancer and diabetes, and he had had an abdominal aneurysm repair surgery at the age of sixty. He was very clear: "No more procedures unless absolutely necessary."

I had to admit I agreed with him. It has now been four years and he remains on the same four blood pressure medications. His kidney function is a little worse but at eighty-two, he is getting by. Interestingly, I heard a story quite similar to Martin's when I attended a session on renal artery hypertension last year at the American Heart Association's annual meeting. The outcome was different, however, because the patient began experiencing episodes of severe fluid buildup in his lungs. This can, in fact, happen in patients with bilateral renal artery stenosis. In such a situation, surgery or angioplasty may relieve the problem. I told Martin about the patient described at the AHA meeting and his response was, "I'll cross that bridge when I get to it." In my opinion this is probably a pretty good approach.

So as you can see, there is no set way to treat renovascular hypertension. At present, there is a great deal of controversy regarding the best approach. If you have renal artery stenosis it will be important to weigh the risks and benefits of all possible treatment strategies with your own physician. In my practice I have found it is crucial to examine each person's situation with an open mind. I would also advise you to seek out the opinion of an expert in the field of hypertension before making a decision regarding a surgical procedure.

PRIMARY ALDOSTERONISM

Secondary hypertension, though uncommon, does occur. Certain causes of secondary hypertension are more common than others. Primary aldosteronism may be as common as renovascular hypertension. Although it is unlikely that the occurrence of primary aldosteronism has increased over the years, what has improved are our techniques for diagnosing this disorder. As a result we are making the diagnosis more frequently.

Laura is a thirty-five-year-old mother of two who had not been to a doctor since the birth of her youngest son seven years ago. She was too busy juggling her job as a stockbroker and her family life to bother taking anyone but her children to the doctor. She felt healthy, ate well, and ran three miles five days a week. She had decided that she could wait until she turned forty for regular check-ups.

But then all of a sudden she began to feel that something was wrong. She had begun having terrible headaches, she was sometimes so fatigued that she missed work (something she had never done in thirteen years), and her muscles had begun to ache.

Over the course of a month, things gradually got worse. Laura was irritable at home, at work she had to fight not to fall asleep at her computer terminal, and daily jogging had become a thing of the past. The first time I met her, she said, "When my husband and kids insisted I see a doctor, I knew things were getting out of hand." She was afraid to make the appointment, knowing that something was radically wrong. She felt certain she must have a brain tumor.

When she finally did call my office, something about her voice made my secretary, Diane, find an appointment where one did not exist. The next day, instead of having lunch I met with Laura. First, Zena, my medical assistant, checked Laura's height, weight, and blood pressure. Her height and weight were perfect, but when Zena found her blood pressure to be 190/110 mmHg, she was certain I would want some blood work done. Before coming to speak to me about it, Zena let Laura relax for a couple of minutes; but the repeat check was no different.

I then ordered a hematocrit (blood count), kidney function, electrolytes (which includes blood sodium and potassium level), blood sugar, and uric acid. I also asked for a cardiogram (EKG) and a urinalysis.

When I met Laura I told her that I thought that her symptoms were related to the high blood pressure reading we had just found. There many things that could cause her blood pressure to be so out of control, but I was confident of being able to get to the bottom of it and she would feel much better soon. This clearly came as a relief to Laura. I warned her that we might have to do a number of tests before a firm diagnosis could be made.

Laura's headaches could be explained just on the basis of her high blood pressure. Her profound fatigue and muscle weakness were not as easily accounted for, but they were probably all related.

I asked Laura about her medical history. Since she hadn't been to a doctor in seven years there was no way to say exactly when the blood pressure problem began (had it been gradual or sudden onset?). It was clear, however, that she had been very healthy. She had been a champion long-distance runner in college, and both her pregnancies had been normal. Her sons, Luke and Colin, ages seven and nine, were healthy. Her parents were in their late fifties and neither had high blood pressure, nor did any of her five brothers and sisters.

Aside from her high blood pressure and overall muscle weakness, her physical exam was normal. I was especially careful to examine her abdomen for "bruits," which you may recall is the word for a sound that results from turbulent blood flow in an artery. When a bruit is heard on an abdominal exam, it can be an indication that there is a blockage in the kidney artery. As discussed previously, such blockages can occur in young women with fibromuscular dysplasia. The fact that I didn't hear a bruit did not eliminate the possibility that Laura had a blockage in her kidney artery, but it did make it less likely.

At the conclusion of the exam, I explained to Laura that her normal physical was encouraging. I started her on Prinivil, an ACE inhibitor, but told her this might not turn out to be the right medication for her. I told her I would likely have more information for her the next day when her laboratory results returned.

The most striking findings on Laura's laboratory studies were her very low potassium level and very high sodium level. These findings in conjunction with her fatigue and muscle weakness made me consider primary aldosteronism.

Primary hyperaldosteronism is a disorder caused by the overproduction of aldosterone from the adrenal glands. The adrenals are very important glands that sit on top of the kidneys. They are divided into two sections, the medulla and the cortex. The cortex consists of three layers. Each layer produces a different type of steroid, and each layer can be involved in some form of secondary hypertension. One of the layers produces aldosterone. This is a steroid responsible for maintaining sodium and potassium balance in the body. Primary aldosteronism can occur in two circumstances. First, it can occur when an adenoma (tumor) develops within the adrenal gland and overproduces aldosterone. Very rarely such tumors can develop outside the adrenal gland. For example, aldosterone-producing tumors have been reported in the ovary. Second, one or both of the adrenal glands can become diffusely enlarged (hyperplasia) and overproduce aldosterone. It is very important to distinguish between an adenoma and hyperplasia because the treatment is different.

At this point my working diagnosis was primary hyperaldosteronism. I explained to Laura that I needed to do a few more laboratory studies. I warned her that if I were right and she did have primary hyperaldosteronism, she would require a CT scan or an MRI and might need surgery as well.

The laboratory studies I ordered were a twenty-four-hour urine collection for sodium and potassium and blood aldosterone and renin levels. If Laura had primary hyperaldosteronism I would expect to find:

- low urine sodium
- high urine potassium
- high blood aldosterone level
- low blood renin level

For this appointment Laura had brought her husband, Jim. He asked why I would expect these particular findings. I explained that the normal function of aldosterone is to cause the kidney to conserve sodium and waste potassium. Normally, when the body is able to produce just the right amount of aldosterone, blood levels of sodium and potassium are perfectly maintained. With excessively high levels of aldosterone in the body, the kidney hangs on to sodium and wastes potassium, and this leads to high blood levels of sodium and very low levels of potassium (both of which we already found in Laura). Potassium is elevated in the urine due to kidney wasting. Sodium is being conserved (held), so very little sodium finds its way into the urine.

The high blood aldosterone level found in primary aldosteronism is the result of overproduction by the adrenal gland. An elevated aldosterone level doesn't help one differentiate between a single adenoma or diffuse hyperplasia, but in the right setting it is helpful in making the diagnosis of primary hyperaldosteronism.

Under normal circumstances the kidney produces renin, which has a crucial role in determining blood pressure. As you have read in this book, renin acts on angiotensinogen in the blood, converting it to angiotensin I, which is ultimately converted to angiotensin II. Angiotensin II has a powerful impact on blood pressure. Renin has other roles as well—it stimulates the adrenal gland to produce aldosterone. When the blood aldosterone level rises dramatically as in primary hyperaldosteronism, renin production is shut down. (The last thing Laura needed would be extra renin, which would further increase the blood level of aldosterone.) So if she did have primary hyperaldosteronism, I would expect that her renin level would be low.

Other studies can be done to help determine if a person has primary hyperaldosteronism. One commonly used test is to measure aldosterone in the urine after a person receives excessive intravenous sodium for three days. Laura was not keen to have such a study so we opted for the blood and urine studies outlined above.

When she was found to have low urine sodium, high urine potassium, an elevated blood aldosterone level, and a very low blood renin level, I was fairly certain that she had primary hyperaldosteronism. In addition, she was the right age and sex for the diagnosis. For reasons unknown, primary aldosteronism occurs twice as often in women as in men and generally strikes between ages thirty and fifty.

I explained to Laura and Jim that the next step should be a spiral CT scan with thin slices through the adrenal glands. This type of CT scan improves the chance of finding even a small adenoma. I prepared Laura and Jim for the fact that if an adenoma were found, I would be recommending surgery. I told them that in my opinion an adenoma would be the best thing to find, because surgery would likely cure Laura's hypertension. If hyperplasia were found, my recommendation would be oral spironolactone therapy.

We were able to schedule the CT scan for the following day. A small right adrenal ademoma was found. Laura and Jim were hoping I would be able to schedule surgery immediately because their children were on summer vacation and both of their jobs were somewhat less demanding during the summer. Laura told me she thought it would be great to recuperate in a lounge chair at the beach. Unfortunately, I had to explain that she would do a lot better with surgery if we treated her high blood pressure for a few months and worked hard to get her body potassium stores back to normal.

Three months later, in mid-October, Laura underwent the successful removal of the adrenal adenoma. She was able to take advantage of the fact that this type of surgery can now be performed using a tiny incision and laparoscopic techniques. A laparoscope is a small instrument with a light source through which surgeons can operate. Many surgeries are now performed using this technique because it results in tiny surgical scars and, more importantly, reduces recovery time. Laura was out of the hospital in three days, back to work in two weeks, and cooking Thanksgiving dinner for twenty-five very thankful people four weeks later. Her only complication was a transient period of very low aldosterone levels.

Today Laura is back to running five days a week, her blood pressure is totally normal, and she feels like herself. At a recent visit Jim commented that their boys both said how glad they were to have their real mother back—the one with too much aldosterone was just too tired all the time. We all laughed to think that at seven and nine aldosterone was in their working vocabulary. Colin, in fact, had done his recent science project on the adrenal gland.

Had hyperplasia been found on Laura's CT scan, spironolactone would have been recommended. Unfortunately, spironolactone therapy can be difficult to tolerate, especially by men, because it can lead to breast enlargement and impotence. Other side effects that can be problematic in both sexes include vomiting, nausea, and fatigue.

Very rarely a person will have a genetic form of primary aldosteronism that is corrected with either steroids or spironolactone. People with this type of primary aldosteronism generally have a strong family history of primary aldosteronism, high blood pressure that develops at a very early age, and family members who have died young of a stroke.

SECONDARY HYPERALDOSTERONISM

It follows that if there is a primary hyperaldosteronism there is also a secondary one. This disorder is generally caused by kidney disease (for example, renal artery stenosis, discussed earlier in this chapter), which leads to excess renin production. High levels of renin in the blood stimulate the adrenal gland to produce aldosterone. People with secondary hyperaldosteronism can be generally distinguished from people with the primary form of the disease because they have high renin levels (those with primary aldosteronism have low renin levels) and because their blood level of potassium is not nearly as low as that seen in primary aldosteronism. Therapy for secondary aldosteronism is directed at the underlying problem, which generally involves the kidney.

HYPERCORTISOLISM: CUSHING'S SYNDROME

The cortex of the adrenal gland is divided into three zones or sections. In our discussion of primary hyperaldosteronism, we reviewed what happens when aldosterone is overproduced. Aldosterone is formed in the zona glomerulosa of the adrenal cortex. Cortisol is another adrenal hormone that is produced in the zona fasciculata of the adrenal cortex. Like excess aldosterone, excess cortisol can also produce hypertension. Cushing's syndrome is the disorder that results from the overproduction of cortisol. It is much more difficult to treat than primary hyperaldosteronism. Thankfully, it is also much less common.

Cushing's syndrome occurs in women three times more commonly than it does in men. In addition, it tends to be a disease of young women, with the diagnosis most commonly being made between the ages of twenty to forty.

Elevated levels of blood cortisol result in a specific array of clinical features. These include truncal obesity (weight gain in the trunk as opposed to the arms, legs, bottom), difficult-to-control high blood pressure (sometimes as high as 200/120 mmHg), a moon face (a visible rounding of the face, often in sharp contrast to the person's previous appearance), fatigue, weakness, depression, osteoporosis (thinning of the bones, especially of the vertebrae in the back), and stretch marks on the abdomen, often with a purplish hue. In addition, women may stop getting their period and have noticeable hair growth on the face and chest.

There are several ways a person can develop Cushing's syndrome. It is crucial to determine its cause, because the therapy for one cause is very different from the therapy for another. Without going into a great deal of detail, normally the pituitary gland (which is found in the head) produces a hormone called adrenocorticotropic hormone (ACTH). This hormone stimulates the adrenal gland to produce cortisol. It stands to reason that a tumor in the pituitary gland that overproduced ACTH would result in elevated blood levels of cortisol and hence Cushing's syndrome.

It is also possible for a tumor in the adrenal gland itself to produce excess cortisol even when the pituitary gland is not overstimulating it. In this case, even in the absence of excess ACTH, blood cortisol levels may be elevated. Finally, certain tumors, most notably lung cancers, produce ACTH and stimulate the adrenal gland to overproduce cortisol. Less commonly, tumors of the ovary and pancreas can produce ACTH, which likewise stimulate the adrenal gland to produce too much cortisol.

In order to determine the exact cause of a person's Cushing's syndrome, a series of tests may be required. If your doctor suspects that you may have it, she will probably first order an "overnight 1 milligram dexamethasone suppression test." Normally dexamethasone, which is a hormone similar to cortisol, will lead to a dramatic reduction in a person's blood cortisol level. If you have Cushing's syndrome, the dexamethasone will not affect your blood cortisol level. In other words, even with 1 milligram of dexamethasone around, the cortisol continues to be pumped out of the adrenal gland.

While the "overnight 1 milligram dexamethasone suppression test" is a good start, some other conditions will result in failure to suppress the blood cortisol level. These conditions include stress, pregnancy, chronic strenuous exercise, some psychiatric conditions, malnutrition, and alcoholism.

If a person fails to suppress cortisol with the "overnight 1 milligram dexamethasone suppression test," the next step is a "low-dose dexamethasone suppression test." This test delivers 2 milligrams of dexamethasone over a period of twenty-four hours. Failure to suppress with this low-dose test means a person has Cushing's syndrome, but it does not help determine the cause (pituitary tumor, adrenal tumor, or other tumor such as of the lung, pancreas, or ovary).

A "high-dose dexamethasone suppression test," which delivers a dose of 8 milligrams of dexamethasone over twenty-four hours, ultimately helps distinguish between pituitary, adrenal, or extra-adrenal (meaning lung, tumor, or other tumor-producing ACTH) cause. By performing the various dexamethasone suppression tests it is possible either to rule out Cushing's syndrome as the cause of the high blood pressure or to determine the most likely cause of the syndrome.

If a person is believed to have Cushing's syndrome as a result of a pituitary tumor, then the next step is magnetic resonance imaging (MRI) of the pituitary. This radiologic procedure allows a good look at the pituitary gland and can find even very small tumors. A pituitary tumor is the most common cause of Cushing's syndrome. If the dexamethasone suppression studies point to the adrenal gland as the most likely culprit, your doctor will order a computerized tomography scan (CT scan) of your adrenal glands to look for a tumor. Finally, if it appears that the ACTH is being produced by an extra-adrenal source such as a tumor, a CT scan of the chest and/or abdomen may be ordered to look for a tumor of the lung, pancreas, or ovary.

Treatment of Cushing's syndrome may involve surgery. While the surgery is being scheduled, the blood pressure is commonly treated with a combination of two types of diuretics. Usual combinations include a thiazide (such as hydrochlorothiazide) and the potassium-sparing diuretic spironolactone.

Once the blood pressure is controlled, a definitive procedure can be undertaken. In general, for pituitary tumors microsurgery is performed. Immediately following surgery, some people experience very low levels of cortisol. This is as dangerous as markedly elevated levels. People undergoing pituitary microsurgery for a tumor are usually given steroid therapy to prevent this occurrence. Because there is a high recurrence rate after pituitary microsurgery, it is crucial to frequently measure cortisol levels following the operation. Children with pituitary tumors are often treated with radiation therapy, and radiation is occasionally used in adults as well. Infrequently, medications such as cyproheptadine, bromocriptine, mitotane, metyrapone, and ketoconazole are used in the treatment of Cushing's syndrome.

Surgical removal of an adrenal tumor can be curative when the tumor is benign. People who have extra-adrenal tumors (lung, ovary, pancreas) resulting in Cushing's syndrome require therapy directed at the underlying tumor. Thankfully, Cushing's syndrome is a very rare cause of secondary hypertension. Should you be diagnosed with it, I recommend that you seek care in a center with special expertise in this disorder.

ENZYME DEFICIENCIES OF THE ADRENAL ZONA RETICULARIS

The third zone of the adrenal cortex is called the zona reticularis. Enzyme defects in this zone can result in multiple signs and symptoms, most appearing in childhood. Two of these enzyme defects (11-alpha and 17-beta hydroxylase deficiency) can result in childhood hypertension. Children with defects of the zona reticularis must be cared for in specialized pediatric centers. Very rarely, a person will have a partial defect in one of these enzymes. In such a case, the high blood pressure might not be recognized until adulthood. People with these enzyme defects are treated with oral steroids, which usually results in a reduction in blood pressure.

PHEOCHROMOCYTOMA

The adrenal gland is composed of two distinctly different parts: the cortex and the medulla. We have just reviewed the hypertensive syndromes that result from defects in the cortex, including hyperaldosteronism, Cushing's syndrome, and 11-alpha and 17-beta hydroxylase deficiency. The adrenal medulla can also be involved in the occurrence of secondary hypertension.

Pheochromocytoma is a very rare but curable cause of secondary hypertension. Depending on the population studied, estimates of the incidence of pheochromocytoma vary from one in every one hundred thousand people per year to one in five hundred thousand people per year. It is safe to say that no matter what the population studied, the condition remains rare.

A pheochromocytoma is an endocrine tumor that secretes mainly catecholamine hormones. These hormones include norepinephrine and epinephrine, as well as a variety of other hormones. Most pheochromocytomas occur in the adrenal medulla but can also develop in extra-adrenal locations, most commonly along the aorta or in the bladder or heart. People with pheochromocytomas can have a variety of symptoms. In large part, symptoms depend on whether the pheochromocytoma is continuously or intermittently secreting hormones and the exact mix of hormones secreted.

About 40 percent of people have a pheochromocytoma that secretes hormones intermittently. These people may experience "spells" anywhere from once a month to daily. Most people with an intermittently secreting tumor experience a "spell" at least once a week. During a "spell," blood pressure can be markedly elevated. Other associated symptoms include sweating, headache, palpitations (racing heart or a sensation of skipped beats) and even a feeling of doom.

Many people say that the spells are totally unpredictable; others note that they can be brought on by activities such as exercise, bending over, urination, defecation, smoking, and even pregnancy. In the case of pregnancy, it is felt that as the uterus enlarges, it may press on the adrenal gland and increase the frequency of the spells. Certain medications, most notably antidepressant/antianxiety medications, can precipitate a spell as can the nicotine in cigarettes.

Many people describe the beginning of a spell in exactly the same way: "All of a sudden I feel a tightness developing in the pit of my stomach. The tightness travels up to my chest and even into my head. I begin to tremble and sweat. My head pounds. I feel as if I might die. Eventually the feeling passes and I am left feeling totally washed out and weak."

Unfortunately, since these symptoms can also occur in an anxiety attack and since anxiety attacks are quite common, many people with a pheochromocytoma are misdiagnosed as having anxiety or depression. They may often be put on an antidepressant/antianxiety medication, which, as noted above, can worsen the situation.

It is estimated that a full 60 percent of people with a pheochromocytoma have continuously secreting pheochromocytomas. They may have intermittent spells in which they experience sweating, palpitations, headaches, and a feeling of doom, but their blood pressure elevation is sustained.

At times a pheochromocytoma may be part of a constellation of endocrine disorders that occur in several members of a particular family. If a person is suspected to have a pheochromocytoma, it is very important to inquire about high blood pressure and endocrine tumors in other family members. The endocrine tumors most frequently associated with pheochromocytomas include those of the thyroid and parathyroid glands as well as tumors of the adrenal cortex. People in families with multiple endocrine tumors should be followed closely for signs and symptoms related to these tumors.

Once a pheochromocytoma is suspected, laboratory studies should be undertaken. The simplest and best screening test is a urine test for the three major products of catecholamine metabolism: metanephrines, free catecholamines (norepinephrine and epinephrine), and vanillylmandelic acid. Sometimes blood catecholamine levels (principally norepinephrine and epinephrine) will be measured.

Although these levels can be useful, sometimes they can be falsely elevated. Salt restriction, vigorous exercise, fasting, smoking, and even upright posture have all been reported to increase blood catecholamine levels. If your doctor suspects you have a pheochromocytoma and wants to check blood catecholamine levels, he will likely do so after you have been lying down with a intravenous catheter in your arm for a few hours. The reason for the intravenous catheter is that blood can be withdrawn without causing you any pain. (Pain can make your catecholamine level climb briefly.)

If the urine test is negative, it is highly unlikely that you have a pheochromocytoma. However, there are rare individuals who only have elevated urinary metabolites of catecholamines immediately following a spell. These people should be supplied with a preservative-containing bottle and instructed to collect a small amount of urine for analysis immediately following a spell. If this too is negative, the person does not have a pheochromocytoma.

If you have a positive urine study indicating that it's very likely that you do have a pheochromocytoma, your doctor will order a CT scan or an MRI of your abdomen to look for the tumor. Typically, pheochromocytomas are easily identified by one of these scans; however, occasionally a person will have a pheochromocytoma that does not show up on an abdominal scan, because it is either very small or outside the abdomen. In such a case, a special radioactive material is injected into the person's vein. This tracer concentrates in the pheochromocytoma, which can then be visualized much more easily.

Once a pheochromocytoma is found, it is crucial to control the blood pressure before performing surgery to remove the tumor. If the blood pressure is not adequately controlled prior to and during surgery, severe complications and even death can result. In general, alpha-blockers are used first, followed by beta-blockers. Most people with a pheochromocytoma are very dehydrated at the time of diagnosis. It is therefore very important to make sure a person has been properly hydrated prior to surgery. If you are diagnosed with a pheochromocytoma, I strongly urge you to have it removed at a center where the surgeon has a great deal of experience with pheochromocytomas. Since this is a rare tumor, you will very likely need to travel to a major medical center for your procedure. The trip is worth it.

Finally, following surgery, many people develop hypoglycemia (low blood sugar). This must be looked for and treated quickly. Most people are cured of their high blood pressure following the surgical removal of the pheochromocytoma, but if blood pressure remains elevated, it is possible that a small amount of the tumor was left behind.

HYPOTHYROIDISM

Hypothyroidism can lead to difficult-to-treat high blood pressure (especially elevations of the diastolic blood pressure), and this appears to be primarily due to an increase in the stiffness of the blood vessels throughout the body. In as many as one-third of patients, treatment of the hypothyroidism with thyroid replacement hormone reverses the high blood pressure. In the other two-thirds, the blood pressure becomes more responsive to traditional blood pressure medications.

If you have very difficult-to-control blood pressure, it is worth asking your doctor to screen you for hypothyroidism. Other symptoms of hypothyroidism include fatigue, dry skin, dry hair, constipation, cold intolerance, and weight gain. Women may note heavy bleeding during their monthly periods. In rare situations a person may experience intellectual decline, hoarse voice, hearing difficulty, and even psychiatric disturbances. Thyroid replacement therapy dramatically improves these symptoms.

HYPERTHYROIDISM

Interestingly, just as hypothyroidism (too little thyroid hormone) can lead to high blood pressure, so to can hyperthyroidism (too much thyroid hormone). People with hyperthyroidism generally come to the doctor complaining of nervousness, difficulty sleeping, excessive sweating, and intolerance of heat. Many also note palpitations, weight loss despite increase in calorie intake, diarrhea, and muscle weakness, and young women frequently lose their periods.

Excess thyroid hormone in the bloodstream speeds up the metabolic rate and causes a hyper-responsiveness to circulating catecholamines. Catecholamines (which include epinephrine and norepinephrine), as you remember from our previous discussion, are naturally occurring chemicals in the bloodstream that help you respond to stressful situations. It is crucial to have some circulating catecholamines, but excessive amounts or hyper-responsiveness to a normal amount of catecholamines can lead to high blood pressure. The treatment of high blood pressure associated with hyperthyroidism generally involves the use of a beta-blocker (e.g., atenolol, propranolol). Not only does this lower blood pressure, but it alleviates some of the other symptoms of hyperthyroidism such as nervousness and palpitations. Depending on the underlying cause of hyperthyroidism, definitive therapy will involve radioactive iodine, propylthiouracil, and sometimes surgery. Once a person has received definitive therapy the beta-blocker may no longer be necessary.

HYPERPARATHYROIDISM

The parathyroid glands sit next to the thyroid gland in the neck. Overproduction of parathyroid hormone due to an adenoma (tumor) in one of the four parathyroid glands can lead to high blood pressure, probably by a number of different mechanisms. Elevations in parathyroid hormone may have a direct effect on the blood vessel, leading to an increase in resistance and hence high blood pressure. In addition, elevated parathyroid hormone leads to an increase in blood calcium level, which can itself lead to high blood pressure.

Most people with hyperparathyroidism are relatively asymptomatic. When symptoms do occur, they are generally the direct result of an elevated blood calcium level. Symptoms include excessive thirst and urination, constipation, thinning of the bones (as calcium leaches out of the bone due to the parathyroid hormone), kidney stones (as calcium overwhelms the kidney's ability to get rid of the excess calcium), and high blood pressure. Treatment involves the surgical removal of the parathyroid gland tumor.

Occasionally, rather than a single tumor in one of the four parathyroid glands the surgeon will discover that all four glands are enlarged. In such a case, 3.5 glands are removed and the patient is followed to determine if the hyperparathyroidism has been cured.

Approximately 10 to 60 percent of people with hyperparathyroidism will have high blood pressure. Unfortunately, while surgery corrects most of the symptoms related to the hyperparathyroidism, most people remain hypertensive even when cured. In some cases, however, the high blood pressure becomes easier to treat.

OBSTRUCTIVE SLEEP APNEA

People who have very difficult-to-control high blood pressure, who snore excessively, have trouble staying awake during the day, and frequently stop breathing for short periods of time during the night should be evaluated for obstructive sleep apnea. The classic person with obstructive sleep apnea is an overweight middle-aged man who drives his bed partner crazy with his snorting, gasping, and snoring. The partner frequently describes periods of apnea (no breathing) followed by gasps.

It is not absolutely clear why people with obstructive sleep apnea have high blood pressure, but it appears that the reduction in blood oxygen associated with the periods of apnea cause the blood pressure to rise. Also people with obstructive sleep apnea seem to lose the normal nocturnal reduction in blood pressure, perhaps because their sleep is so fragmented.

If obstructive sleep apnea is suspected, it is crucial to perform an all-night sleep study in a sleep laboratory, as this is a potentially curable cause of refractory hypertension. When both high blood pressure and excessive daytime drowsiness are evident, most sleep specialists consider the finding of five to fifteen episodes of apnea due to obstruction of the airway per hour of sleep to be diagnostic for obstructive sleep apnea.

Obstructive sleep apnea may be cured with weight loss and restriction of substances (such as alcohol) that decrease respiration and increase snoring. In some patients, underlying medical conditions such as hypothyroidism may contribute to the development of the syndrome, and in such cases, treatment of the underlying medical condition may correct the sleep apnea.

Some people will require more complex therapies such as nasal CPAP (continuous positive airway pressure)—facial appliances to prevent the tongue from obstructing the airway or surgery. The use of nasal CPAP involves the delivery of oxygen in a continuous fashion through a face mask. This therapy is often effective in reducing daytime drowsiness and improving blood pressure. The downside of nasal CPAP is that the mask itself is quite bulky and can be uncomfortable to wear while sleeping. Other devices move the tongue in such a way as to prevent obstruction of the airway. These devices suffer from the same problem as nasal CPAP, namely, it can be difficult to find a comfortable sleep position. Finally, some people will undergo a surgical procedure called a uvulopalatopharyngoplasty. This procedure removes obstructive neck tissue, and when successful can markedly improve blood pressure, symptoms, and snoring.

MORBID OBESITY

Most overweight individuals can be managed with standard blood pressure–lowering medications. There are, however, some overweight people who respond very poorly to traditional blood pressure medications. After extensive evaluation of such a person it generally becomes clear that it is his obesity that is responsible for a failure to respond adequately to medications. Weight loss efforts are essential, but some people cannot diet effectively because they have a pathological relationship with food.

In some cases weight loss medications or psychological evaluation and treatment may be helpful. However, for some people heroic measures such as gastric bypass surgery are clearly necessary. It should be pointed out that even gastric bypass can fail if a person is unwilling to make the necessary dietary changes.

Over the last ten years I have referred three patients (two men and one woman) for gastric bypass surgery. Each was taking four blood pressure medications with only marginal control of his or her blood pressure; and in each case, as the individual had gained weight over the years, the blood pressure had become more and more difficult to control.

I met Drew at the time of his first heart attack. At six feet tall he weighed 260 pounds (his ideal weight would be about 180). His blood pressure on two blood pressure medications was 140/90. In addition, he had high cholesterol and a borderline blood sugar. My initial hope was that with weight loss his blood pressure, cholesterol, and blood sugar would all improve. I was hopeful that having had a heart attack would motivate him to make lifestyle changes.

At first things went beautifully. Drew lost 15 pounds, his blood pressure dropped, his cholesterol improved (although he did require a cholesterol-lowering medication), and his blood sugar fell into the normal range. This lasted for about six months. Suddenly Drew lost all his motivation. My guess is that the previous six months had been driven by fear of a second heart attack. The further away Drew got from his heart attack, the less motivated he became. Over the next three years no matter what I tried or how many times he saw our nutritionist, he kept gaining weight. Three years after his heart attack Drew weighed 300 pounds, and he was on four blood pressure medications at high doses. He was also on two cholesterol medications and a single medication to lower his blood sugar.

Although I was fairly certain I would not find a secondary cause for his refractory high blood pressure, we ruled out most of the causes described earlier in this chapter. When it was crystal clear that weight was the cause of Drew's high blood pressure, I broached the idea of gastric bypass surgery. At first Drew refused even to consider the procedure, saying he felt that was just giving in—he should be able to conquer his compulsive eating. When we looked at his history, however, we found that since high school he had gained 100 pounds and had never been successful at keeping weight off long-term. He had been on every fad diet ever on the market: pills, shakes, and prepackaged diet foods. Nothing had worked. Finally he agreed to let me describe the procedure.

I explained that a gastric bypass involves constructing a small pouch which is connected between the esophagus and the intestines. Food travels from the esophagus into the pouch and then into the intestine, bypassing the stomach. The pouch serves as a person's "new stomach." Because of its small size, the pouch allows a person to feel full quickly and with a small amount of food. The surgery is very important, but will only be successful when combined with behavioral modification.

Drew's surgery went without a hitch, but it took him about six months to feel fully recovered. He attended a behavior modification program at our center and began a daily walking program. Gradually over the first year Drew lost 100 pounds. His weight stayed stable at 200 for about six months, then he increased his walking and lost another 10 pounds. He doesn't think it is likely he will get much below 190 pounds, but as far as I am concerned, he is doing just fine. He is currently on just one blood pressure medication (a beta-blocker), and he no longer requires medications to lower his cholesterol or blood sugar levels.

Most important is the fact that Drew feels much better about himself. He told me that in the past he spent so much time thinking about his weight that it colored everything he did and all his personal relationships. He told me that his weight loss dramatically improved his self-confidence. In fact, he finally had the confidence to apply for a promotion in his company. When he went to the corporate headquarters, the interviewer asked Drew why, with his qualifications, he had not applied for a promotion sooner. Drew told him that the timing had not been right previously, but that he felt he was now ready and would do a great job. He immediately got the job and a huge raise.

Drew also confided that he has a much better relationship with his wife and sons. None of his three boys are overweight and all are very athletic, something Drew had always been very proud of. He attended all their games and cheered them on. Although the boys never said anything, Drew feels sure that as he lost weight they became more pleased to have him at their games. Drew told me that one of his proudest moments since his gastric bypass came when his youngest son asked him to coach his basketball team. Drew has said more than once that he wonders why he waited so long to have the gastric bypass. My feeling is, he did it at just the right time.

CHAPTER 10

≈∫

HYPERTENSION IN SPECIAL POPULATIONS

Throughout this book I have commented on other diseases or medical issues that might influence your doctor's decisions regarding how best to treat your high blood pressure. In this chapter I will address these issues in an orderly and systematic way, so you will be able to use this information as a quick reference. I will discuss treating high blood pressure in these special cases:

- A person with heart disease
- A person with Syndrome X (insulin resistance, high cholesterol and high blood pressure) or with diabetes
- A person with high cholesterol
- A person with cerebrovascular disease—(stroke or transient ischemic attack)
- A person with peripheral vascular disease
- Pregnant women
- Children and adolescents
- The elderly

Noticeably absent from this list is a person with kidney disease. People with significant kidney disease frequently have difficult-to-treat hypertension and almost always require medications. This topic was covered in full in chapter 9, so it will not be repeated here.

HEART DISEASE

If you have heart disease and high blood pressure it is important that your doctor consider both when making treatment decisions. Failure to do so could mean a missed opportunity for choosing a medication with the ability to treat both conditions. It could also spell disaster: Certain medications may be great at lowering blood pressure in a person with a healthy heart, but have negative effects on a person with underlying heart disease.

In terms of lifestyle changes, you will be encouraged to restrict salt and increase potassium and calcium in your diet. If you need to lose weight, you should follow a low-fat, low-cholesterol diet. (See chapter 5.) Although exercise is certainly desirable, it is very important that you take proper precautions before beginning any new program. As a cardiac patient, you may eventually develop a very vigorous running, swimming, or walking regime, but you should never start without first getting the approval of your doctor.

In general, I recommend that cardiac patients with high blood pressure start with a supervised cardiac rehabilitation program, generally beginning with a stress test. During a stress test you walk/run on a treadmill while hooked up to electrodes that record cardiac function. A stress test allows your physician to evaluate the function and health of your heart while you are exercising. In turn, your physician will be able to set exercise limits for you. As you become stronger, the exercise prescription can be modified. Having an exercise prescription gives you the confidence you need to make sensible decisions about when to push yourself and when to relax.

Even if lifestyle changes alone totally normalize your blood pressure, if you also have heart disease there is still good reason to take blood pressure–lowering medications. In some cases the medication is being used to protect the heart and reduce the risk of future heart attacks (as in certain beta-blockers, calcium channel blockers, and ACE inhibitors). In other situations medications that lower blood pressure are used because of their ability to minimize episodes of chest pain, also known as angina. Drugs that reduce angina include beta-blockers, calcium channel blockers, and nitrates.

Certain agents should clearly be avoided by people who have both high blood pressure and heart disease. These include direct vasodilators such as Apresoline (hydralazine) and Loniten (minoxidil). Although these are excellent blood pressure–lowering medications and are typically used in people with highly resistant blood pressure, they cause the heart rate to speed up. This increase in heart rate is undesirable because it can result in severe ischemia (inadequate oxygen supply to the heart muscle). This same phenomenon has been observed when people with high blood pressure and heart disease are treated with Procardia or Adalat (nifedipine). Interestingly, however, if a person has a particular type of heart disease characterized by spasm of the heart arteries, then nifedipine may be just the right choice.

How will your doctor decide what medication is right for you if you have heart disease and you also require blood pressure medication? By heart disease I mean you have angina, or have had a heart attack, an angioplasty, or bypass surgery. Like me, your doctor will turn to the literature and look at the evidence from available clinical trials. One very important publication is *The Sixth Report of the Joint National Committee on Prevention, Detection, Evaluation, and Treatment of High Blood Pressure* (JNC VI). Since 1988, hundreds of experts in the field of hypertension have worked together to publish six reports (each adding new information based on available clinical trials), which provide physicians nationwide with up-to-date recommendations on the best treatment options in a wide variety of situations.

In the case of a person with heart disease and high blood pressure the *JNC* VI clearly recommends beta-blockers as the first-line agents. They specifically recommend the class of beta-blockers that have been shown in clinical trials to reduce the risk of a future heart attack or sudden cardiac death. Beta-blockers falling into this group include Tenormin (atenolol), Toprol or Lopressor (metoprolol), Corgard (nadolol), or Inderal (propranolol).

The *JNC* VI goes on to recommend ACE inhibitors, especially if a person has experienced heart failure following his heart attack. Since the publication of the *JNC* VI in 1997, a very important trial called the Heart Outcomes Preventive Evaluation (HOPE) trial, including over 9,000 patients, was published in *The New England Journal of Medicine*). The HOPE trial found that the ACE inhibitor Altace (ramipril) could dramatically reduce the risk of a heart event (by 22 percent) even if a person did not have a history of heart failure.

For a person who is unable to tolerate either a beta-blocker or an ACE inhibitor, there are several good alternatives. Isoptin SR, Calan SR, Veralen or Covera HS (verapamil) or Cardizem SR, Cardizem CD, Dilacor XR, Tiazac (diltiazem) are good choices; they have been shown to reduce cardiac events in the face of a heart attack uncomplicated by heart failure—a person whose heart is still able to squeeze properly with each heartbeat. These calcium channel blockers are known as nondihydropyridines.

The European Trial of Systemic Hypertension in the Elderly (Syst-Eur) utilized a dihydropyridine calcium channel blocker called nitrendipine, which at the present time is available only in Europe. In this trial, this agent dramatically reduced the risks of stroke and heart attack. Based on these data, it might be acceptable to consider the use of Norvasc (amlodipine), one of the currently available dihydropyridines, for a person with a history of heart disease.

Many people who have heart disease and high blood pressure will require more than one medication to normalize blood pressure. When combination therapy is needed, good pairs include a beta-blocker in combination with an ACE inhibitor, or a beta-blocker in combination with a calcium channel blocker. In the latter case, note that the dihydropyridine calcium channel blockers such as Norvasc (amlodipine) are safer in combination with a beta-blocker than are the nondihyropyridine calcium channel blockers such as verapamil and diltiazem. The concern when one of the nondihyropyridines (especially verapamil) is combined with a beta-blocker is the risk of developing a dramatic reduction in heart rate (complete heart block). This can be a life-threatening situation.

Finally, nitroglycerin, which is often placed under the tongue to relieve cardiac chest pain, is also available in long-acting preparations. Although not often thought of as a blood pressure–lowering medication, long-acting nitrates can in fact have a substantial blood pressure–lowering impact.

You might also wonder what your goal blood pressure should be in the face of high blood pressure and a history of heart disease. In the past people have been concerned that lowering blood pressure too dramatically might cause chest pain and ischemia (inadequate blood flow/oxygen delivery to the heart cells). In order to address this issue, the Hypertensive Optimal Treatment (HOT) Study was undertaken. Involving just under 19,000 patients, this study found that in people with heart disease, the optimal blood pressure appeared to be 138/83 mmHg. Importantly, no worsening of angina or heart outcomes was observed in participants if their diastolic blood pressure was lowered further, even down to the 70 mmHg range.

SYNDROME X OR DIABETES

In the late 1980s, Dr. Gerald Reaven, who was then the director of the Division of Endocrinology and Metabolism at Stanford University School of Medicine, noted that high blood pressure, glucose intolerance (or insulin resistance), high triglycerides, and low HDL (good) cholesterol often occurred together in a single person. He called this constellation of findings Syndrome X.

The terms *glucose intolerance* or *insulin resistance* deserve an explanation. In a person without insulin resistance, the blood glucose (sugar) level rises after eating a meal. This triggers the pancreas to secrete the hormone insulin. One of insulin's functions is to cause sugar in the bloodstream to move into the cells, where it is used for energy, thus maintaining a healthy blood sugar level.

A person with glucose intolerance or insulin resistance is still able to move sugar into the cells, but with great difficulty. In this situation, the pancreas must make a lot of extra insulin to successfully lower the blood sugar. Although technically people with insulin resistance do not have blood sugar levels high enough to diagnose diabetes (>126 mg/dl), their levels are not totally normal and tend to hover between 110 and 126 mg/dl in the fasting state.

From a metabolic point of view elevated insulin levels and high triglycerides go hand in hand. Insulin not only promotes the movement of sugar into the cells, it also prevents fat cells from releasing fatty acids into the bloodstream. People who are insulin resistant tend to have fat cells that release fatty acids into the bloodstream to a much greater extent do people who are not insulin resistant. These fatty acids travel to the liver, where they are used as fuel to produce triglycerides. Triglycerides are a blood fat, which tends to be elevated in people who are overweight and sedentary. Interestingly, these are the same conditions we see in people with insulin resistance. There is no doubt that people with high triglycerides are at increased risk of the development of heart disease and stroke.

There is also a direct metabolic relationship between triglycerides and HDL-cholesterol—the higher the triglycerides, the lower the HDL-cholesterol. It should not be surprising that people who have Syndrome X tend to have low HDL-cholesterol. In multiple clinical studies, low HDL has been shown to predict the development of early heart disease.

You may be asking yourself why it is so important to know about Syndrome X. It should not come as a surprise that people with Syndrome X are at very high risk of the development of future heart disease. Dr. Reaven published the results of two clinical trials, one in the *Journal of Clinical Endocrinology and Metabolism* in 1998 and the other in *Metabolism* in 1999. The first study looked at 147 middle-aged men and women who were considered healthy at the start of the study. Participants were divided into three groups according to levels of insulin resistance, and these individuals were followed for five years. Of those who were most insulin resistant, one out of seven experienced a heart attack during the follow-up period. In the group that had the lowest levels of insulin resistance, no one had a heart attack.

In the second and larger study, 650 participants were divided into four groups from least to most insulin resistant. This time the groups were followed for ten years. Eight percent of the people with the greatest insulin resistance had a heart attack during the follow-up period, whereas only 1 percent of the least insulin resistant did. This is not a new finding. In 1996, *The New England Journal of Medicine* published the Quebec Cardiovascular Study, whose results were strikingly similar.

It is important to note that Syndrome X has both a genetic component and an environmental one. By this I mean that there is no doubt that some of us are more likely, based on our genes, to develop Syndrome X. However, being genetically predisposed to Syndrome X and actually developing it are two different things. If you are genetically predisposed you can push things along by being sedentary and gaining weight. On the other hand, exercise and if necessary weight loss can stall or prevent the development of Syndrome X.

If you have Syndrome X, developing an exercise program can go a long way toward improving blood pressure, HDL-cholesterol, triglycerides, and insulin resistance. After a complete discussion and approval from your doctor, I suggest you aim to develop the walking program outlined in chapter 4.

Weight loss also dramatically improves all the metabolic derangements seen in people with Syndrome X. Although the standard low-fat diet outlined in chapter 5 will promote weight loss, we often advocate a slightly higher fat and lower carbohydrate diet in the treatment of Syndrome X. In such a case, we recommend the monounsaturated fats as the best choice. These include canola, olive, and peanut oils. We also suggest the judicious use of small amounts of almonds, walnuts, pistachios, filberts, and peanuts.

As you increase your intake of fat, it is crucial for you to also reduce your intake of carbohydrate. Remember that fat is very calorie dense (9 calories per gram) as compared to carbohydrate and protein (4 calories per gram). In a diet that contains a greater percentage of fat, the absolute amount of food you are allowed will necessarily be somewhat less.

For women on the Syndrome X diet we suggest 1,200 calories and up to 40 grams of fat (that is, 360 calories from fat); in other words, 30 percent of calories come from fat. For men we suggest 1,500 calories and 50 grams of fat (450 calories from fat). Again, this is a diet in which 30 percent of calories come from fat. Some people have gone as far as advocating up to 40 percent of calories from fat. When it comes to losing weight, we find that people do better on the 30 percent fat program.

If you require a medication for your blood pressure and you have Syndrome X, there is some evidence that the ACE inhibitor Altace (ramipril) can reduce the likelihood of your developing diabetes.

In the past, the alpha-blockers were recommended because of their ability to improve insulin resistance. This is certainly still true, but the alpha-blockers have recently fallen out of favor as first-line blood pressure medications, in large part due to their less than stellar performance in the ALLHAT trial. (See chapter 7.)

In people who already have diabetes, it is important to note that in the United States, diabetes and high blood pressure are the two most common causes of kidney failure requiring dialysis.

Just having diabetes has been shown to dramatically increase the risk of heart disease. In 1998, *The New England Journal of Medicine* published Dr. Steven Haffner's East-West Study. This study found that over the course of seven years a person with diabetes but no history of a heart attack is at the same risk of having a heart attack as is a person who has already had one. And the risk is very high— approximately 20 percent in the diabetic group and 19 percent in those with a previous heart attack.

If, on top of diabetes, you add high blood pressure, the risk increases still further. It follows that treating the high blood pressure in a person with diabetes is likely to reduce risk. The question is, how low should the blood pressure be lowered? It appears that the lower, the better. Reducing the pressure to less than 140/90 mmHg has certainly been shown to reduce both progression of kidney disease and the need for dialysis. Likewise, it has been shown to reduce cardiovascular events. Lowering the pressure to less than 130/85 mmHg is even better.

Achieving a blood pressure below 130/85 mmHg often means taking two and even three blood pressure medications. Which drugs are used in combination can have a great deal of impact on how well the pressure is lowered and how commonly side effects are experienced.

Because the ACE inhibitors have the most favorable impact on progression of kidney disease, they should (if tolerated) be used as a first-line drug for diabetics with high blood pressure. If the ACE inhibitors are not tolerated (likely because of a dry cough, which can develop in up to 10 percent of people taking the drug), then one should consider the angiotensin receptor blockers. Although less data are available on the angiotensin receptor blockers, it does appear that they will have the same favorable effects on kidney function. If a second agent is required, a good case can be made for the nondihydropyridine calcium channel blockers such as verapamil or diltiazem. These agents have been shown to have some impact (although less complete than the ACE inhibitors) on stalling the progression of kidney disease. At times, especially if a person with diabetes and high blood pressure has significant leg and ankle edema (fluid buildup), a diuretic is a better second choice than is the calcium channel blocker.

People with significant kidney disease (commonly those with diabetes) frequently have blood pressure that is extraordinarily difficult to control. In such cases, very strong blood pressure medications such as minoxidil (combined with a beta-blocker and a strong diuretic) may be required. This combination can have a dramatic impact on blood pressure, but note that both beta-blockers and diuretics can worsen diabetes control, while minoxidil has some potentially negative effects on kidney function. Nonetheless, on occasion, this combination can forestall the need for dialysis.

If you have diabetes and high blood pressure, it is crucial to work closely with your doctor on controlling these and all other cardiac risk factors. It is quite common for diabetics also to have cholesterol problems (especially high triglycerides and low HDL-cholesterol). Ask your doctor to check your fasting cholesterol profile. As noted previously, I cannot emphasize enough the importance of diet, exercise, and weight loss.

HIGH CHOLESTEROL

If you have both high blood pressure and high cholesterol, you are at high risk of developing heart disease and stroke. In the 316,000 men who were screened for the Multiple Risk Factor Intervention Trial (MRFIT), these two risk factors were synergistic—the risk associated with having both high blood pressure and high cholesterol was greater than the sum of the risk of having either condition alone. It is very common for a person with high blood pressure to have high cholesterol too.

How do you know if you have high cholesterol? In order to measure your blood cholesterol level accurately you will need to

Table 10.1 Normal Blood Fat Levels

BLOOD FAT	DESIRABLE LEVEL
Total cholesterol[1]	< 200 mg/dl (if no CAD)[2]
	< 150 mg/dl (if CAD)
Triglycerides	< 150 mg/dl (if no CAD)
	< 100 mg/dl (if CAD)
LDL-cholesterol	< 130 mg/dl (if no CAD)
	< 100 mg/dl (if CAD)
	Ideal < 80 mg/dl (if CAD)
HDL-cholesterol	> 45 mg/dl

[1]**The total cholesterol is really the composite of the triglycerides/5 + LDL + HDL.**

[2]**CAD = coronary artery disease (generally defined as having had a heart attack, bypass, angioplasty, or an abnormal stress test indicating heart disease). Other disorders considered to be coronary artery disease equivalents are peripheral vascular disease (blockages in the leg arteries), cerebrovascular disease (blockages in the arteries leading to the brain), and diabetes. A person with one of these conditions is at high risk of having a vascular event (heart attack, stroke, etc.) and thus should take a very aggressive approach to cholesterol reduction.**

fast for twelve hours. A more complete picture of your cholesterol profile is obtained if you are fasting. Once you have your cholesterol levels back you can use Table 10.1 to determine if you have a problem with any of the blood fats.

The triglycerides are a blood fat that tends to rise in the face of alcohol intake, increased weight, a diet rich in sugar and fat, and a sedentary lifestyle. There is no doubt that elevated triglycerides increase the risk of developing heart disease and stroke. It has been shown that people who have high triglycerides also tend to have elevations in blood pressure and increased risk of developing diabetes. It follows that the way to lower your triglycerides is to cut back on alcohol, exercise daily, restrict sugar and fat in your diet, and lose weight if necessary. If these measures fail, your doctor may prescribe a triglyceride-lowering medication such as Tricor, Lopid, or Niaspan.

LDL-cholesterol stands for low-density lipoprotein cholesterol. You have probably heard of the "good and bad cholesterol." LDL-cholesterol is the "bad cholesterol." Elevated levels of LDL-cholesterol dramatically increase a person's risk of heart disease and stroke. LDL-cholesterol sticks to the artery wall and over time can cause blockages to develop.

Most people who have a heart attack do not have a complete blockage of the heart artery when the attack occurs. Rather, the cholesterol plaque (blockage), which contains large amounts of LDL-cholesterol, can become unstable. This may cause the plaque to crack open. When this happens within an artery, the body's natural response is to try to repair the area with a blood clot. The combination of a cholesterol plaque and a blood clot can spell disaster. If the artery is totally blocked, a heart attack will occur. LDL-cholesterol is high in people with certain genetic abnormalities and in people who have a diet rich in saturated fat. If LDL-cholesterol is a problem for you, it is important to restrict dietary fat (especially saturated and hydrogenated fats). Likewise, losing weight will help lower your LDL-cholesterol. Finally, if these measures fail, your doctor may prescribe one of the so-called statin medications (Lipitor, Zocor, Baycol, Mevacor, Lescol, or Pravachol).

The HDL-cholesterol (which stands for high density lipoprotein cholesterol) is also known as the "good cholesterol." The role of HDL-cholesterol is to bring the bad cholesterol back to the liver for processing. People with high levels of this type of cholesterol appear to be protected against heart disease. Of course, a person can have an excellent HDL-cholesterol level and still develop heart disease, especially when he also has other risk factors such as high blood pressure, diabetes, and cigarette smoking.

In large part a person's HDL-cholesterol level is genetically pre-determined (meaning your level really depends on the genes your parents have given you). There are, however, some things you can do to improve your HDL-cholesterol level. Quitting smoking can increase your HDL-cholesterol level by as much as 8 mg/dl. Generally the full impact is seen within six months of quitting.

Exercise is also known to improve HDL-cholesterol. Men tend to get a greater increase during the first year (as much as 10 percent), but if women keep at it, studies have shown as much as a 20 percent improvement. Weight loss can lead to a significant improvement in this lipoprotein, but often as a person is actively losing weight the HDL-cholesterol level will transiently decline. Don't get discouraged if this happens to you. Once you reach a new weight plateau your HDL level will increase and ultimately exceed your old level. Finally, if you require more HDL improvement than the aforementioned hygienic measures can provide, your doctor may prescribe Niaspan, Lopid, or Tricor.

By now it should be pretty obvious that the lifestyle measures that will improve your cholesterol profile are the same ones that will improve your blood pressure: weight loss, regular exercise, quitting smoking, and eating a healthy diet rich in fruits and vegetables and low in fat.

As your physician works with you to lower both your blood pressure and your cholesterol, he must carefully assess your medications. In chapter 2 I noted that some medications can lead to high blood pressure. The same is true regarding high cholesterol. Table 10.2 reviews the impact of some commonly used medications.

You may wonder what some of these medications are or what they are used for. Amiodorone (Cordarone, Pacerone) is used to treat certain heart arrhythmias. Androgens, such as Android capsules or Testoderm, are used frequently to treat testosterone insufficiency in men, or certain cancers in women.

Table 10.2 Effects of Medication on Triglycerides and Cholesterol

	TRIGLYCERIDES	LDL	HDL
Amiodarone	increase	increase	
Androgens			reduce
Beta-blockers	increase		reduce
Cyclosporin	increase	increase	
Progestins		increase	reduce
Protease inhibitors	increase		
Retinoids	increase	increase	reduce
Steroids	increase	increase	increase
Diuretics	increase	increase	

Beta-blockers, as noted earlier in this book, are blood pressure medications. Not all beta-blockers adversely affect cholesterol. Most notably, acebutolol (Sectral), carteolol (Cartrol), carvedilol (Coreg), celiprolol (Selectrol), penbutolol (Levatol), and pindolol (Visken) are the beta-blockers that do not have an adverse impact on lipids. On the other hand, the most commonly used beta-blockers including atenolol (Tenormin), metoprolol (Lopressor, Toprol), nadolol (Corgard), and propranolol (Inderal) all adversely affect blood lipid levels. In one Veterans Administration study, propranolol increased triglycerides by 42 mg/dl. It should be noted, however, that the beta-blockers with an adverse impact are actually the group of beta-blockers shown to protect against recurrent heart attack in people who have already suffered one. For this reason, it is sometimes essential to use a beta-blocker and work around the adverse impact on lipids.

Cyclosporin (Neoral, Sandimmune) is an immunosuppressive agent used in people who have undergone a heart or kidney transplant. For these people the drug is irreplaceable and its impact on blood lipids must be dealt with.

Progestins are one of the components of most birth control pills and are used as part of postmenopausal hormone replacement therapy. In general, the goal is to use the lowest possible dose of a progestin. In the case of birth control pills, the agents that have the least negative impact on the cholesterol profile include Ortho Tri-Cyclen, Modicon, and Brevicon. When progestins (such as Cycrin, Provera, Prometrium capsules) are used as part of the post-menopausal hormone regime the goal is to use the lowest possible dose. In the Postmenopausal Estrogen Progestin Intervention (PEPI) Trial the progestin with the least negative impact on the lipoprotein profile was micronized progestin (Prometrium is an example of micronized progestin).

Protease inhibitors such as Crixivan, Agenerase capsules, Fortovase, Invirase, Norvir, and Viracept have dramatically improved the lives of people with HIV/AIDS, but like most things, they come with a price. People on the protease inhibitors experience a marked increase in blood lipids, most notably a dramatic increase in triglycerides. For most of these people the protease inhibitors simply cannot be discontinued. In general, people on these agents require a lipid-altering agent. Because both protease inhibitors and lipid-altering medications can adversely affect liver function, it is crucial to follow patients taking both agents very closely.

Retinoids such as Accutane are used in the treatment of cystic acne. Thankfully most people on Accutane are teenagers who use it for brief periods of time. Although lipids can be dramatically altered, levels typically revert to normal following therapy.

Steroids such as prednisone are frequently used for short periods in the treatment of poison ivy or for an attack of asthma. If a person's exposure to poison ivy or asthma attacks are infrequent, the negative impact on the lipid profile presents little worry. Unfortunately, there are many people on chronic steroids for a host of rheumatologic disorders, for severe asthma, for chronic lung disorders, and to prevent rejection of transplanted organs. For these people the adverse impact on lipids will require careful management. A person who will require lifelong steroids must take the lowest possible dose. In some cases it is possible to use steroid-sparing medications (i.e., a medication that will allow the use of a lower dose of a steroid).

Finally, diuretics, another blood pressure–lowering medication, can markedly alter the cholesterol profile. Again, in some cases they are absolutely necessary. Remember that indapamide (Lozol) is one diuretic that has very little negative impact on cholesterol levels.

If one of the above medications appears to be the culprit in your high cholesterol, your doctor may want to alter your medications in hopes of improving your cholesterol. If at all possible, avoid beta-blockers and diuretics known to adversely affect lipids. If a medication is needed to treat your high blood pressure and you have high cholesterol, I favor using a drug that is lipid neutral (meaning it does not have any impact on cholesterol levels). Drugs in this category include ACE inhibitors, angiotensin II receptor blockers, and calcium channel blockers. In the past I would often recommend the alpha-blockers to treat high blood pressure in people with high cholesterol. My reasoning was simply that the alpha-blockers could lower cholesterol as they lowered blood pressure.

As mentioned earlier in this book, the very large ALLHAT trial found that Cardura, an alpha-blocker, actually increased the risk of cardiac events as compared to the diuretic chlorthalidone. For this reason the Cardura portion of the ALLHAT was discontinued early. I no longer routinely prescribe the alpha-blockers as first-line therapy for high blood pressure. They may, however, have a role as a second agent in a person whose blood pressure is not adequately controlled with just one.

Finally, it is interesting to note that medications for the treatment of high cholesterol have also been shown to lower blood pressure. In the September/October issue of the journal *Hypertension*,

Glorioso published a study showing that the cholesterol-lowering medication Pravachol (pravastatin) lowered both systolic (8 mmHg) and diastolic (by 5 mmHg) blood pressure as well as lowering the LDL-cholesterol.

CEREBROVASCULAR DISEASE

Cerebrovascular disease is the third-leading cause of death in the United States. Roughly 500,000 Americans will suffer a stroke this year and almost a third of them will die from it. Currently almost four million Americans have suffered stroke. Stroke can rob a person of the ability to work, to live independently, or to speak or walk. Many of my patients tell me that they fear a stroke much more than they fear a heart attack or even death.

Approximately 85 percent of strokes are due to cerebral infarction. This occurs when there is an interruption in the supply of blood to the brain. The other 15 percent of strokes are due to hemorrhage. In both situations high blood pressure is a major risk factor.

There is little doubt that high blood pressure dramatically increases the risk of developing a stroke, so it is only logical to think that excellent control of blood pressure should be the goal for a person with high blood pressure. Likewise, one would have to surmise that aggressive control of blood pressure would be the order of the day for a person who has recovered from a stroke. Unfortunately, the data available to guide physicians on how aggressive to be with blood pressure control is scant. When it comes to the studies on how to treat blood pressure in the face of an acute stroke, even less information is available.

Although there are not a great many studies on the impact of hypertension control on the subsequent risk of developing stroke, there are a few. The Systolic Hypertension in the Elderly Program (SHEP) proved that using a diuretic to treat hypertension could result in a marked reduction in stroke. More recently the Systolic

Hypertension in Europe (Syst-Eur) study used the dihydropyridine calcium channel blocker, nitrendipine, and found a 42 percent reduction in stroke.

Sometimes a person may have no symptoms of cerebrovascular disease, but on physical exam a bruit (French for "sound") is heard. When a person has a partial blockage of one of the carotid arteries (the two arteries found in the front of your neck on either side of the thyroid gland), a bruit can be heard through a stethoscope. If the carotid artery has a partial blockage, blood traveling to the brain through the artery encounters it and resulting blood flow becomes turbulent, creating a whooshing sound (a bruit). If a bruit is found on physical exam, an ultrasound of the artery is undertaken to determine the extent of vascular disease. Depending on the size and other features of the blockage, carotid surgery (carotid endarterectomy) may be recommended.

In general, if a person has asymptomatic carotid artery disease, whether she undergoes surgery or not, aggressive reduction of blood pressure is recommended. It is also recommended that people who have recovered from a stroke and those at high risk of developing cerebrovascular disease should be treated aggressively. Although the goal blood pressure has not been established, most authorities would agree that it should be somewhat below 125/85 mmHg.

On the other hand, it may be appropriate to be less forceful with a person who has high-grade blockages in his carotid arteries. The concern here is that a rapid or dramatic reduction in blood pressure might further compromise an already tenuous blood flow to the brain. For these people, a gradual reduction to 140/90 mmHg prior to carotid surgery might be appropriate.

A stroke is truly the most feared complication of high blood pressure. It is likely that almost everyone reading this book has a friend or family member who has suffered a stroke. In the time that I have been writing this book, two of my aunts have died of strokes (Aunt Sheila and Aunt Rita). Both were wonderful people who had very difficult-to-control high blood pressure, and both of them died too soon.

If you have a family member or close friend who has suffered a stroke, chances are you have gone to the hospital to visit. And you may have been surprised, and possibly worried, when you saw that your loved one's blood pressure was quite high and that little was being done about it.

Unfortunately, when it comes to determining the optimal blood pressure during and immediately following a stroke, there are almost no studies to guide treatment practices. Sometimes, just as for a heart attack, clot-dissolving medications are used to dissolve blood clots that have caused the stroke. Anytime a "clot-buster" such as tissue plasminogen activator or TPA is given, there is a risk of causing bleeding in the brain. In such a case, a person's stroke would get much worse instead of better. Experience has taught us that the higher a person's blood pressure when he arrives at the hospital with a stroke, the greater the risk of bleeding if TPA is given. For this reason, TPA, which can be lifesaving and can dramatically reduce the severity of a stroke, is reserved for people whose systolic blood pressure is less than 185 mmHg and diastolic below 110 mmHg. On occasion TPA is given when a person's systolic blood pressure is between 185 and 220 mmHg, but clearly this places him at high risk of complications.

Sometimes blood pressure is so high during a stroke that intravenous medications such as nitroprusside are needed. Nitroprusside is a potent vasodilator, typically used in the face of a diastolic blood pressure greater than 140 mmHg. When the systolic blood pressure rises above 220 mmHg, intravenous labetalol, an alpha-beta-blocker, is used. Because of the concern that a stroke may be worsened by reducing blood pressure, and therefore blood flow to the brain, no specific blood pressure medications are recommended if the systolic blood pressure is 185–220 mmHg or the diastolic blood pressure is between 105 and 120 mmHg. This reluctance to use medications after an acute stroke may be modified in the face of other complicating circumstances. For example, if a person with an acute stroke develops kidney failure, a heart attack, or an aortic dissection (see chapter 7), blood pressure reduction is warranted.

As noted at the beginning of this section, not all strokes are caused by cerebral infarction. Roughly 15 percent are caused by hemorrhage. Once again the optimal blood pressure goal in the acute setting is not absolutely certain. In general, medications to lower blood pressure are reserved for people whose systolic blood pressure is above 180 mmHg and/or diastolic blood pressure is above 140 mmHg. Just as is the case with a cerebral infarction, the medications chosen to lower blood pressure include intravenous sodium nitroprusside, labetalol, and enalapril.

Once a person has stabilized, it is necessary to attend to careful blood pressure reduction. In general, the blood pressure is gradually lowered to 140/90 mmHg. The ultimate goal is a blood pressure less than 125/85 mmHg. Care must be taken to lower blood pressure gradually. Failure to do so may result in the development of side effects such as dizziness and confusion.

The same lifestyle recommendations for lowering blood pressure apply in the poststroke setting as in the absence of a stroke: weight loss, a low-fat diet rich in fruits and vegetables (good sources of potassium) and low in salt, giving up smoking, and starting an exercise program.

Which medication to use for blood pressure reduction following a stroke is generally guided by other medical conditions. For example, a person who has both heart disease and cerebrovascular disease should be on a beta-blocker and/or an ACE inhibitor because these agents not only reduce blood pressure but also protect against further heart disease. In this situation a case could also be made for a calcium channel blocker.

Following a stroke, a person who has diabetes or kidney disease will likely benefit from an ACE inhibitor. As noted earlier, in the absence of other medical conditions, which might push your physician to choose one of the above mentioned agents, diuretics and dihydropyridine calcium channel blockers have been shown to reduce the risk of stroke in large clinical trials.

Finally, note that two classes of cholesterol-lowering medications, the statins and fibric acid derivatives, have both been shown to lower the risk of stroke by between 19 and 30 percent. The statins include drugs such as Lipitor, Zocor, Baycol, Pravachol, Mevacor, and Lescol and the currently available fibric acid derivatives include Lopid and Tricor.

PERIPHERAL VASCULAR DISEASE

Peripheral vascular disease (PVD) is caused by atherosclerosis in the lower extremities. The most common symptom associated with PVD is leg pain known as intermittent claudication. Although it is not always the case, most people with intermittent claudication know exactly how far they can walk before developing leg pain. Some people with claudication describe days when they can walk much further. Even on good days, however, these people are limited. The pain associated with intermittent claudication is not always confined to the legs, but can extend to the thighs and even hips. Universally, rest relieves the pain and the resumption of walking makes it recur.

Most available data suggest that the major risk factors for the development of peripheral vascular disease are cigarette smoking, diabetes, and high blood pressure. When it comes to high blood pressure, elevated systolic (the pressure in the body's arteries when blood is pumping out of the heart) rather than diastolic blood pressure is more tightly linked to the development of PVD. The higher the systolic blood pressure, the more likely PVD is to develop.

There is surprisingly little data regarding whether or not treating hypertension in a person with PVD actually slows its progression. In the Treatment of Mild Hypertension Study (TOMHS), aggressive treatment of high blood pressure with lifestyle changes and medications did prevent the development of intermittent claudication.

Once again lifestyle changes can result in improvement in both blood pressure and walking distance for people who already have PVD and are troubled by intermittent claudication. Developing a daily walking program is crucial. Your doctor will be able to guide you, but typically the recommendation is walking to the point of pain, resting, and doing it again. The goal is to walk a total of forty-five minutes a day. This may take quite some time to achieve. Even if you are unable to reach the forty-five minute mark, any exercise is better than none. In the words of Dr. Peter Wood from Stanford University, "People get their biggest benefit just from getting off the couch." After your doctor's approval you can use the walking program outlined in chapter 4.

Quitting smoking is another crucial lifestyle change. Quitting smoking has been absolutely proven to increase walking distance, and since blood pressure rises with each cigarette smoked, the ups and downs will be minimized.

You might wonder how your doctor goes about picking a medication if you suffer from both high blood pressure and PVD. One recent study suggested that the blood pressure lowering–calcium channel blocker, verapamil, may increase the distance a person is able to walk before experiencing claudication. Likewise, ACE inhibitors have been claimed to improve walking distance as well as blood pressure. There is, of course, no doubt that the ACE inhibitors do lower blood pressure; however, there is really very little data to support the claim that they improve walking distance.

Some studies have concluded that beta-blockers worsen PVD. Careful analysis of these studies has not borne this claim out. Nonetheless, when I start a person with PVD on a beta-blocker, I am careful to point out that there is a possibility that their PVD may worsen. I ask them to contact me immediately if this occurs.

Unfortunately then, with the possible benefits associated with verapamil, there really are no blood pressure medications that stand out as improving both PVD and blood pressure simultaneously. This is not the case for lifestyle; both exercise and quitting smoking can provide benefits in both arenas.

PREGNANCY

High blood pressure during pregnancy can be very serious and potentially life threatening. On the other hand, women who have had mild or moderately high blood pressure prior to becoming pregnant may actually experience a drop in blood pressure during the second trimester of pregnancy. In this situation it may actually be possible to withdraw blood pressure medications and monitor closely.

A new development of high blood pressure during pregnancy (in a woman who previously had normal or even low blood pressure) is entirely different from the continuation of high blood pressure in a woman who has had it for a long time. Since the development of high blood pressure during pregnancy can be life threatening we will discuss this situation, also known as preeclampsia (which can progress to eclampsia) first. This will be followed by a discussion of the treatment of chronic high blood pressure during pregnancy.

Preeclampsia is a hypertensive condition unique to pregnancy. Despite the fact that the condition has been described for centuries, the cause of preeclampsia remains a mystery. There are multiple theories regarding the underlying cause, but no definitive proof for any of them.

One theory suggests that the preeclamptic placenta is abnormal in its blood supply system and therefore produces certain cytokines (chemicals found in the blood, often in response to infection or injury) and hormones, which result in high blood pressure in the mother. In this theory the abnormal placenta is the cause rather than the result of the condition.

Other theories center on abnormalities in the mother's body. People who espouse this point of view note that although overall preeclampsia complicates roughly 3 percent of all pregnancies in the

United States (7 percent of first pregnancies), certain women are at much higher risk than others. For example, up to 25 percent of women with diabetes, chronic high blood pressure, underlying kidney disease, or a history of previous preeclampsia will develop preeclampsia.

Interestingly, women bearing twins are also at very high risk of developing preeclampsia. At somewhat lower but still increased risk are women with genetically high cholesterol, clotting abnormalities, and high blood levels of homocysteine (an amino acid we all have in our blood). Finally, still other scientists point to an interaction between the mother and the placenta as the cause of preeclampsia.

One very interesting finding is that preeclampsia occurs more commonly in a first pregnancy than it does in subsequent pregnancies, as long as the father is the same. If a woman has multiple pregnancies with different partners, her risk remains high for each pregnancy; but in multiple pregnancies with the same partner, the risk, although still high, drops considerably. This finding suggests that preeclampsia might be triggered in part by an inflammatory response to something in the father's sperm and that continued exposure reduces the response.

What are the signs and symptoms of preeclampsia? In general, it complicates a first pregnancy more than any other. Things may have been totally uneventful for the first two trimesters, and then (typically sometime early in the third trimester), a previously normotensive young woman will develop blood pressure greater than 140/90 mmHg. If a woman previously had high blood pressure, preeclampsia should be suspected when the blood pressure climbs by 30 mmHg (systolic) or 15 mmHg (diastolic). Other associated findings include protein in the urine, as well as swelling of the face, hands, and ankles. Abnormalities in laboratory tests including blood count, platelets (the cells responsible for blood clotting), and blood chemistry (especially liver function, uric acid and albumin) can be dramatic.

The greatest concerns is that she will go on to develop either the HELLP syndrome (Hemolysis, which is the destruction of blood cells, Elevated Liver function tests, and Low Platelets) or eclampsia, which is the life-threatening end result of preeclampsia. While there may be little warning before a woman proceeds from preeclampsia to HELLP, prior to developing eclampsia many women with preeclampsia experience changes in their reflexes and vision, severe headaches, and abdominal pain (especially in the upper right-hand area of the abdomen).

The only definitive treatment for preeclampsia, HELLP, and eclampsia is delivery of the baby. In general almost immediately after delivery, blood pressure and laboratory findings return to normal. This may sound very reassuring, but the major worry is making sure that a healthy baby is delivered to a healthy mother. The goal is always to extend the pregnancy as long as possible (at the very least to thirty-two, but hopefully to thirty-six weeks). Since preeclampsia almost never resolves on its own (i.e., without delivery), the goal is stabilization as opposed to cure. The two most important therapies currently employed for stabilization are bed rest and intravenous magnesium sulfate. The bed rest tends to lower blood pressure just by virtue of inactivity and the magnesium sulfate prevents seizures.

Why not just treat women who are at high risk for preeclampsia (i.e., women with diabetes, kidney disease, high blood pressure, genetically high cholesterol, clotting abnormalities, high homocysteine, and twins) with something to prevent its development? This is a great thought, but unfortunately thus far treating with aspirin or calcium supplements have been unsuccessful. Theoretically, both of these therapies make sense, but theory and practice are not always the same thing.

You might also wonder why we don't just treat women with preeclampsia with blood pressure medications. This is actually a very controversial subject. The major concern is that if blood pressure is lowered too much, it might lead to sluggish blood flow both to the placenta and to the developing infant. It is also clear that blood pressure medications do not in any way alter the progression of preeclampsia to eclampsia.

Accordingly, when blood pressure medications are given to a woman with preeclampsia they are given solely for maternal safety. However, it is true that if blood pressure can be controlled, it may mean that the mother will be able to remain pregnant longer and her infant will continue to grow and develop. The National Institutes of Health Working Group on Hypertension in Pregnancy recommends medications when the diastolic blood pressure is above 100 mmHg.

Medication choices will differ depending on when delivery is expected, with the intravenous medication hydralazine being used most commonly when delivery is imminent. If it appears that delivery may be days or even weeks away, methyldopa remains the drug of choice. Sometimes beta-blockers, combination alpha-beta-blockers, or even long-acting calcium channel blockers are chosen for a woman who has side effects from methyldopa.

The treatment of a woman with long-standing high blood pressure who becomes pregnant is quite different from the treatment of a woman who develops preeclampsia during pregnancy. It should be pointed out that since women with preexisting high blood pressure are at somewhat increased risk of developing preeclampsia during pregnancy, a goal of all hypertensive women wishing to become pregnant should be normalization of blood pressure with lifestyle changes.

When a hypertensive woman contemplating pregnancy asks me what she might be able to do to improve her chances of a healthy pregnancy, I ask about her lifestyle. We discuss weight loss (if this is indicated), initiation of a low-impact aerobic exercise program, salt restriction, increased potassium, and calcium intake. I also recommend folic acid supplementation. If she is drinking alcohol I suggest she stop, both to reduce the risk of fetal alcohol syndrome (the leading cause of mental retardation in the United States) should she become pregnant quickly, and also as a means of lowering blood pressure.

Not every woman will be able to normalize her blood pressure with lifestyle changes alone, but most women with high blood pressure should be able to have a successful and uneventful pregnancy. It is important for women with high blood pressure to have frequent evaluations throughout their pregnancies. And because the risk of preeclampsia is higher in women with underlying high blood pressure, careful monitoring for evidence of its development is essential.

Interestingly, blood pressure tends to decline during the second trimester of pregnancy. Sometimes women who are on blood pressure medications can reduce their dose or even discontinue their medications at this time.

For women already on drug therapy, it may be necessary to switch to an alternate medication. A drug that may be just fine for a nonpregnant woman may not be the right choice during pregnancy. Unfortunately, very few medications have been carefully evaluated in pregnant women.

You can understand the dilemma. You certainly don't want to expose a woman to a medication that might harm her unborn baby. On the other hand, if a woman has markedly elevated blood pressure it needs to be treated. Because there were few choices for blood pressure reduction thirty to forty years ago, the drugs that were around were commonly used. Later beta-blockers and alpha-beta-blockers were also used. Although not always free of side effects, these drugs have been found to be relatively safe for both mother and child. Methyldopa does, however, have the potential for two serious side effects: liver disease and a rare anemia called Coombs-positive hemolytic anemia. Fortunately, both of these side effects are rare. Beta-blockers are generally well tolerated, but may lead to smaller babies.

Under no circumstances should ACE inhibitors or angiotensin receptor blockers be used during pregnancy. The concern is that these drugs can cause severe kidney failure in babies whose mothers take them, especially in the last two trimesters of pregnancy. So little is known regarding the use of calcium channel blockers in pregnant women that they are best avoided.

Finally, because blood pressure medications can get into breast milk, generally speaking breastfeeding is not recommended for women who must be on a blood pressure medication. If a woman feels strongly about breast feeding and has borderline blood pressure levels, it is probably acceptable to allow her to breast feed for a few months before initiating blood pressure medication.

In summary, pregnancy may be associated with some serious and sometimes life-threatening blood pressure problems. With very careful monitoring even women with preeclampsia can deliver healthy babies. Good prenatal care is essential for all women, but especially for women with preexisting hypertension and women at increased risk of developing preeclampsia. When choosing a medication to control blood pressure during pregnancy, it is important to keep in mind both the mother and her unborn baby.

CHILDREN AND ADOLESCENTS

A full discussion of the diagnosis and treatment of high blood pressure in childhood is beyond the scope of this book. Nonetheless, a few comments must be made. One of the most important reasons for including a discussion on children and adolescents is because many of you reading this book have children. A child whose parents have high blood pressure is at much higher risk of developing it himself as compared to a child whose parents are normotensive (even if both children have identical blood pressure readings). Recognizing that your children do not live in a genetic vacuum, but rather share your genes, may make you more vigilant about their salt and potassium intake, physical activity, and weight.

Starting at the age of three, when your child goes to the doctor for her yearly physical, a blood pressure measurement should be obtained. Unlike adults, for whom a high reading is considered greater than 140/90 mmHg, the definition of high for children varies according to age, sex, and height. Your child's pediatrician will use the chart in Table 10.3 from the National High Blood Pressure Education Program Working Group on Hypertension in Children and Adolescents, published in *Pediatrics* in 1996. The levels shown indicate the ninety-fifth percentile of blood pressure for boys and girls ages three to sixteen based on height. Levels at or above the ninety-fifth percentile are considered high blood pressure. Levels above the ninetieth percentile are not depicted but are considered high normal and warrant close follow-up. In general the ninetieth percentile is 4 mmHg lower than the ninety-fifth percentile reading.

Many factors predict which children with high normal or high blood pressure will become adults with high blood pressure. The most important is a family history of high blood pressure and obesity. In children with high blood pressure, at least 50 percent have a family history of high blood pressure in a first-degree adult relative. Some studies have found that obese children are more responsive to salt in the diet (meaning more likely to experience an increase in blood pressure) than are normal weight children. Likewise African American children frequently are hyper-responsive to salt when compared to their white American peers. This is not dissimilar to the findings regarding salt sensitivity differences in African American adults and white American adults.

Some investigators have wondered whether the correlation between family history has more to do with shared genetics or the shared environment of the parent and child. It would be natural to

Table 10.3 Normal Blood Pressure in Children

BLOOD PRESSURE	AGE	HEIGHT PERCENTILE FOR GIRLS				HEIGHT PERCENTILE FOR BOYS			
		5th	25th	75th	95th	5th	25th	75th	95th
Systolic	3	104	105	108	110	104	107	111	113
	6	108	110	112	114	109	112	115	117
	10	116	117	120	122	114	117	121	123
	13	121	123	126	128	121	124	128	130
	16	125	127	130	132	129	132	136	138
Diastolic	3	65	65	67	68	63	64	66	67
	6	71	72	73	75	72	73	75	76
	10	77	77	79	80	77	79	80	82
	13	80	81	82	84	79	81	83	84
	16	83	83	85	86	83	84	86	87

examine adopted children to help answer this question. Genetics appears to be a very powerful predictor as there is a stronger correlation between biological parent and child than adoptive parent and child.

No matter what the genetic issues, parents can still work to provide their children with an environment that will reduce the likelihood of their developing high blood pressure either in childhood or later life. Such an environment provides the child with ample physical activity and a diet rich in fruits, vegetables, and calcium. The optimal diet is also low in salt and saturated fat. It should provide enough calories to promote healthy growth and development, but avoid excessive calories that can cause obesity.

A child who gains 10 pounds over the course of a single year (unless she has grown two or more inches) should be monitored closely to prevent the development of obesity. At the present time, the United States is faced with a record number of overweight or obese children. Twenty-five percent of children and adolescents in the United States are either overweight or obese. If we do not do something to correct this, we are poised for a virtual explosion of high blood pressure in the next generation.

Just like adults, some children have secondary causes for their high blood pressure. In general, the higher the blood pressure and the younger the child, the more likely it is that a secondary cause of high blood pressure will be found. Such a cause is almost always of renal (kidney) origin. The second most common cause of secondary high blood pressure in children is something called coarctation of the aorta, which is caused when a narrowing occurs in this blood vessel. The narrowing results in a normal blood supply to the upper body and a diminished blood supply to the lower body. Children with coarctation of the aorta will have diminished pulses in the legs and are often noted to have high blood pressure. Since surgery is curative it is essential to make this diagnosis. It is also important to make the diagnosis promptly because the earlier surgery is done (generally when a child is about a year old) the better the outcome.

In general, if there is a secondary cause of high blood pressure in a child or adolescent, it will be detected by the following battery of tests:

A family history: Do any relatives have high blood pressure and if so, has an underlying secondary cause been identified?

A personal history: Is this child taking any medications known to raise blood pressure such as nonsteroidal anti–inflammatory medications? Does this child or adolescent use street drugs (amphetamines or cocaine)? Has this child had multiple urinary tract infections that might cause scarring of the kidneys?

A dietary assessment, especially with regard to calories, salt, and potassium intake

A physical exam: height, weight, blood pressure (taken in both the arms and legs), pulses throughout the body, evaluation of the eyes, heart, and abdomen

A laboratory evaluation: urinalysis, complete blood count, kidney function, blood electrolytes (sodium and potassium are of special interest), cholesterol levels

Other studies may include an echocardiogram, which is an ultrasound study that can evaluate the size of the heart, how well the walls of the heart move, and the movement of the heart valves. Only rarely are additional studies, typically of the kidney (for example, a kidney ultrasound or evaluation of the kidney arteries) deemed necessary.

The treatment of children with high blood pressure usually focuses on lifestyle changes, although in some cases medications are needed. In general, diuretics and beta-blockers have been the mainstays of drug therapy. Over the last few years there is growing evidence that the ACE inhibitors and calcium channel blockers are safe for children. It must be remembered, however, that ACE inhibitors are not recommended during pregnancy. Since many adolescent girls become pregnant, great caution must be exercised in prescribing an ACE inhibitor for a teenage girl with high blood pressure.

A complete discussion of the aforementioned medications can be found in chapter 7.

OLDER PEOPLE

There are a number of reasons for including a separate section on the treatment of high blood pressure in older people. First, in the past people have wondered if it is worthwhile to treat high blood pressure in the older population. The point has been: "What good will it do? They have to die of something—why not heart disease or stroke?" (This argument has always seemed particularly hard-hearted and actually not very sound.)

Second, there is clear evidence that aging can change the rate at which medications are metabolized. In many cases this means that lower doses of blood pressure medications will achieve good blood pressure control. It can also mean that certain side effects can be more pronounced in the elderly. Last but certainly not least, whereas many young working people have insurance coverage for their blood pressure medications, many older, retired people must pay out of pocket. I find that drug costs for older people living on a fixed income must be a major consideration as I decide on medications for my patients.

To address the first issue, "What good will it do?" I first point out that more cardiac events and strokes occur in older people than any other population in the country. These events don't just kill people, they can leave them with severe disabilities and markedly reduce their quality of life. Aside from this purely cold and analytic perspective, there have now been four major clinical trials in older populations (generally defined as over sixty or sixty-five), which have proven that blood pressure reduction in this population dramatically reduces the risk of heart attack or stroke. These studies have been carried out in both the United States and Europe and include the Systolic Hypertension in the Elderly Program (SHEP), the Swedish Trial in Old Patients with Hypertension (STOP–1), the Medical Research Council Elderly Trial (MRC-E), and the European Trial on Isolated Systolic Hypertension (SYST-EUR).

In terms of the second issue, as people age there are changes in the liver blood flow and kidney function. Since these are the two main organs for drug metabolism, these changes will have a significant impact on a person's ability to metabolize many medications. The end result is that a medication at a certain dose may have a very different impact in an older versus a younger person. For example, the dose of a drug that provides perfect blood pressure control in a younger person may lower it profoundly with a prolonged effect in an older person. In some cases this can be used to an older person's advantage (cutting a pill in half or taking it less frequently may mean a less expensive treatment plan). On the other hand, it can be problematic, because a slow metabolism of some drugs can result in an increased risk of side effects. These can include dizziness and severe hypotension. These symptoms can occur frequently when an older person takes a diuretic (water pill) and fails to drink a sufficient amount of water.

It appears that older people are more troubled by the constipating effects of verapamil than are younger people. In part this is due to the fact that many of them are on other constipating medications as well, and the additive impact of these medications can be very troublesome. One thing you can do if you become constipated while taking a blood pressure medication is to increase your intake of water and exercise more. Both help decrease the constipation and may allow you to continue taking an otherwise excellent blood pressure–lowering medication.

In chapter 7 I mention that the ACE inhibitors can cause a cough in up to 10 percent of people who use them. Unfortunately, the cough seems to occur somewhat more frequently in the elderly, especially in women.

If you are over sixty and your doctor suggests a blood pressure medication, it is important to discuss her plans for the starting dose and dose titration.

As your doctor decides which medication is right for you, he is likely to look to the clinical trials and ask which blood pressure medications have been proven to work in the elderly. It is equally important to consider other medical problems you may have. Some medications will improve or worsen other medical problems. Since we all tend to "collect" more medical problems as we age, this is a very important consideration. It is crucial for the doctor to know your medical history well. It doesn't hurt for you to be well informed, either.

In the clinical trials that have included older people, thiazide diuretics, chlorthalidone (also a diuretic), and the dihydropyridine calcium channel blocker nitrendipine have all been shown to reduce the risk of heart attack or stroke. Because of this "hard" data, the current national guidelines recommend diuretics as first-line therapy for blood pressure control in the elderly. The calcium channel blocker nitrendipine is not available in the United States. Norvasc (amlodipine), another dihydropyridine, is available in the United States. Accordingly Norvasc should be considered a good choice for treating hypertension in this population.

Remember that the national guidelines are just that—guidelines. Your doctor may have a good reason for choosing an alternative medication. If you have high blood pressure and heart disease, your doctor is likely to choose a beta-blocker. Based on recent clinical trials, an ACE inhibitor such as Altace (ramipril) would be another excellent choice. Other trials have suggested that the nondihydropyridine calcium channel blockers may also protect against recurrent heart attacks.

If you have kidney disease, heart failure, or diabetes, it is likely that an ACE inhibitor will be used as part of your blood pressure treatment plan. Beta-blockers have also been shown to benefit people with heart failure and may be chosen in this situation both for their blood pressure–lowering effect and their ability to reduce symptoms and effects of heart failure. People with arthritis may require nonsteroidal anti-inflammatory medications such as Motrin or Nuprin. It is well known that in the face of the anti-inflammatory medications, blood pressure medications work less well. The only exceptions to this rule are calcium channel blockers, which work just as well when a person is taking a nonsteroidal.

Osteoporosis (thinning of the bones) is a very common problem in older women and makes fractures a distinct possibility. Since a hip fracture can mean the loss of living independently for many women, it is important to note that diuretics have been shown to improve bone mass. Having greater bone mass may mean fewer fractures.

Ethnic background also makes a difference in medication selection for older people. One study performed by the government found beta-blockers and ACE inhibitors were the best choice for overall blood pressure reduction in whites over the age of sixty, while calcium channel blockers and diuretics performed better in older blacks.

In summary, it is important for your doctor to take into account your age and your other medical problems as she decides what medication is best for you.

Epilogue

꒒

I hope you have enjoyed this book. I know it got a little complex in places, but this couldn't be helped. Hypertension is a complex subject, and I felt that you deserved to know everything your doctor knows about the subject. After all, it is your body—and you are the person with high blood pressure. Hopefully, you are now also the person who has his or her blood pressure under perfect control.

I hope you found that the information outlined in this book helped you identify changes that you can make in your lifestyle. As you make these changes, remember that you are reworking old habits, and old habits die hard—that's why they call them habits! If you slip up with your diet, exercise, or alcohol intake—or if you smoke a cigarette—don't be too hard on yourself. Most of all, don't give up. Carefully examine what happened and identify a plan to prevent it from happening again. You can do it!

Many people tell me that they feel like a failure if they require a blood pressure medication. However, if you are genetically predisposed, or if you require medications (for other illnesses) that have blood pressure elevation as a side effect, blood pressure–lowering medications will be required no matter how good you are with lifestyle. If you need a medication, please take it faithfully. It may save your life.

As I mentioned in the preface of this book, for people with high blood pressure, the future has never looked so good. But it's in your hands. Use the information you have learned in this book and decide today to live a long and healthy life.

Glossary

ACE inhibitors (angiotensin-converting enzyme inhibitors).
A class of blood pressure–lowering medications. These agents are especially useful for people with heart disease, diabetes, or kidney disease. Examples include: benazepril (Lotensin), captopril (Capoten), enalapril (Vasotec), fosinopril (Monopril), lisinopril (Prinivil, Zestril), moexipril (Univasc), quinapril (Accupril), ramipril (Altace), and trandolapril (Mavik). (See chapter 7 for a full discussion of ACE inhibitors.)

Adrenaline. A hormone produced by the adrenal gland. This hormone is also known as epinephrine and is produced at times of fright, excitement, or anger.

Adrenocorticotropic hormone (ACTH). A hormone produced by the pituitary gland, which stimulates the adrenal gland to produce the hormone cortisol.

Aerobic exercise. Exercise in which the muscles utilize oxygen (aerobic means "with oxygen") to burn both sugar and body fat. Examples include walking, running, swimming, skiing, and cycling.

Aldosterone. A hormone produced by the adrenal gland, which promotes salt and water retention. Excess levels of aldosterone in the bloodstream can cause high blood pressure.

Alpha-adrenergic blockers. A class of blood pressure–lowering medications that block alpha-receptors. Examples include: doxazosin (Cardura), prazosin (Minipress), terazosin (Hytrin). (For a complete discussion of alpha-adrenergic blockers see chapter 7.)

Alpha–beta–receptor antagonists. A class of blood pressure–lowering medications that work by blocking both alpha and beta receptors. Examples include: labetalol (Normodyne, Trandate) and carvedilol (Coreg). (For a complete discussion of alpha–beta–receptor antagonists see chapter 7.)

Ambulatory blood pressure monitor. A blood pressure monitor that is worn for a period of twenty-four hours, during which time it automatically inflates at preset time intervals. Blood pressure levels are recorded and stored within the device for review.

Amiodarone (Cordarone, Pacerone). A drug used to treat heart arrhythmias, which can cause cholesterol and thyroid abnormalities.

Anaerobic exercise. Exercise that is performed in short intense bursts and that does not utilize oxygen. Examples include weight lifting and sprinting.

Androgen. A male hormone.

Aneurysm. A bulging out of the muscular wall of a blood vessel or heart. It occurs at a weak point and is the result of disease or injury. Untreated high blood pressure can cause a weakening or aneurysm in the aorta (our most important blood vessel). If an aneurysm ruptures or bursts death may occur.

Angina pectoris. Chest pain or pressure resulting from insufficient blood flow (and oxygen delivery) to the heart muscle—typically, the result of blockages within the coronary arteries. In some people angina is felt as arm, jaw, or neck pain.

Angioplasty. See *Coronary artery balloon angioplasty.*

Angiotensin I. A physiologically inactive form of angiotensinogen. Angiotensin I is converted by the action of angiotensin-converting enzyme (ACE) to angiotensin II, a strong vasoconstrictor of blood vessels.

Angiotensin II. A strong vasoconstrictor. Excess amounts of angiotensin II can lead to high blood pressure.

Angiotensinogen. A protein produced by the liver, which is converted to angiotensin I when acted upon by renin (a chemical produced in the kidney).

Angiotensin-receptor antagonists (sartans). A new class of blood pressure–lowering medications that block the ability of angiotensin II to cause vasoconstriction. Examples include: losartan (Cozaar), valsartan (Diovan), and irbesartan (Avapro). (For a full discussion of the angiotensin-receptor antagonists see chapter 7.)

Anti-anginal. A drug that relieves symptoms of angina (chest pressure, back pain, jaw pain, shortness of breath).

Antihypertensive. A medication that lowers blood pressure.

Aorta. The most important artery in the body. This blood vessel carries blood away from the left side of the heart. Many blood vessels including the coronary arteries spring from the aorta.

Arrhythmia. An electrical disturbance in the heart rhythm that is often the result of underlying coronary artery disease.

Arteries. Blood vessels that carry oxygenated blood away from the heart to the rest of the body. The only exception is the pulmonary artery, which carries oxygen-poor blood to the lungs from the right side of the heart.

Atherosclerosis. A disease process that begins in childhood, characterized by the gradual buildup of plaque within the artery wall. Hypertension is a major risk factor in the development of atherosclerosis. Other risk factors include elevated cholesterol, cigarette smoking, diabetes, obesity, sedentary lifestyle. Cholesterol is the major constituent of the plaque. When a plaque becomes unstable, it can rupture and lead to angina or a heart attack.

Baycol. A cholesterol-lowering medication.

Beta-blocker. A medication used to treat high blood pressure. Beta-blockers are also used in the treatment of angina and reduce the risk of heart attack. Some beta-blockers cause blood triglycerides to rise and the

HDL-cholesterol (the protective cholesterol) to fall. Beta-blockers can also lead to an increase in blood sugar. Examples include: acebutolol (Sectral), atenolol (Tenormin), betaxolol (Kerlone), bisprolol (Zebeta), carteolol (Cartrol), carvedilol (Coreg), celiprolol (Selectrol), labetalol (Normodyne, Trandate), metoprolol (Lopressor, Toprol XL), nadolol (Corgard), penbutolol (Levatol), pindolol (Visken), propranolol (Inderal, Inderal LA), timolol (Blocadren). (See chapter 7 for a full discussion of beta-blockers.)

Body mass index (BMI). A measure of obesity calculated by dividing a person's weight in kilograms by height in meters squared.

Bruit. French for "sound," it refers to the sound heard in an artery with a partial cholesterol blockage.

Bupropion (Wellbutrin, Zyban). An antidepressant medication that is also used in smoking cessation.

Bypass. See *Coronary artery bypass grafting.*

Calcium channel blocker. A type of medication used to treat high blood pressure. Calcium channel blockers are also used to treat angina and may reduce the risk of heart attack. Examples include: amlodipine (Norvasc), felodipine (Pendil), isradipine (DynaCirc), nicardipine (Cardene SR), nifedipine (Procardia XL, Adalat), nisoldipine (Sular), verapamil (Isoptin SR, Calan SR, Verelen, Covera HS), diltiazem (Cardizem SR, Cardizem CD, Dilacor XR, Tiazac). (See chapter 7 for a full discussion of calcium channel blockers.)

Cardiac. Pertaining to the heart.

Cardiac catheterization. See *Coronary angiography.*

Cardiac rehabilitation program. A thrice weekly, medically supervised exercise program attended by people with cardiac disease. Such programs also generally include advice on diet, smoking cessation, and stress reduction.

Cardiac risk factors. Aspects of one's life that predispose to the development of cardiac disease. These include: elevated high blood pressure, cholesterol, smoking, diabetes, family history of heart disease, obesity, a sedentary lifestyle, stress, elevated blood homocysteine, elevated lipoprotein (a), and elevated C-reactive protein, as well as being a male over the age of forty-five, or being a postmenopausal female.

Carotid arteries. Arteries in the neck that arise from the aorta and carry blood to the brain.

Carotid endarterectomy. A surgical procedure performed when the carotid arteries are occluded with cholesterol plaque.

Catheterization. See *Coronary angiography.*

Central sympatholytics. A class of blood pressure–lowering medications that work by blocking the sympathetic nervous system in the brain. Examples include: clonidine (Catapres), guanabenz (Wytensin), guanfacine (Tenex), methyldopa (Aldomet). (For a full discussion of central sympatholytics see chapter 7.)

Cerebrovascular. Pertaining to the blood vessels serving the brain.

Cerebrovascular disease. Blockages in the blood vessels serving the brain, which can result in stroke.

Cholesterol. A white waxy substance found only in products of animal origin, including egg yolks, meat, cheese, milk, and ice cream. Cholesterol is also produced by all the cells of the body, especially by the liver cells. Small amounts are necessary to make cell walls and hormones.

Claudication. Pain in the lower extremities resulting from inadequate circulation.

Coronary angiography. A procedure in which dye is injected into the coronary arteries via a flexible catheter (a thin, hollow plastic tube) to determine if these arteries have significant blockages.

Coronary artery. An artery that supplies blood and oxygen to the heart muscle. Coronary arteries arise from the aorta. The major arteries include the right coronary artery and the left main artery, which quickly divides into the circumflex and left anterior descending arteries.

Coronary artery balloon angioplasty. A procedure in which a thin catheter containing an inflatable balloon is used to open a blocked artery. A metal stent is often placed in the artery at the site of the blockage to prevent the artery from closing following an angioplasty.

Coronary artery bypass grafting. Open heart surgery in which a leg vein (saphenous vein) or breast artery (mammary artery) is used to connect the aorta with a coronary artery just beyond a blockage.

Coronary artery disease (CAD). A progressive disorder caused by blockages in the coronary arteries. Aftereffects of this disease include angina pectoris, heart attack, and sudden cardiac death. Individuals with CAD require lifestyle changes and risk factor reduction, and may require coronary artery bypass grafting or angioplasty.

Cyclosporin (Neoral, Sandimmune). A drug that prevents rejection in people who have had an organ transplant. This agent can cause high blood pressure.

DASH (Dietary Approaches to Stop Hypertension) Trial. A blood pressure trial conducted in the late 1990s to determine if a diet rich in fruits and vegetables might reduce blood pressure.

Dexamethasone suppression test. A study during which a person is given the hormone dexamethasone. Under normal circumstances this hormone causes the adrenal gland to temporarily cease (suppress) the production of cortisol. Failure of the adrenal gland to cease production can indicate an underlying problem with either the adrenal or pituitary glands.

Dexfenfluramine (Redux). A weight loss medication that was taken off the market in the late 1990s due to valvular heart disease and the potential deadly side effect of primary pulmonary hypertension (a restrictive lung disease).

Diabetes. A condition in which repeated fasting blood sugar levels are above 126 mg/dl.

Dialysis. A procedure used in kidney failure to maintain electrolyte balance and to remove wastes and toxins from the blood. Hemodialysis is performed in a specialized center three times a week. Continuous ambulatory peritoneal dialysis (CAPD) is an alternative to hemodialysis performed by the person with kidney failure. CAPD involves instilling fluid into the abdominal cavity for several hours; the fluid is then drained, taking with it waste fluids and toxins.

Diastolic blood pressure. The pressure in the body's arteries between heartbeats (as the heart is filling with oxygen-rich blood returning from the lungs).

Direct vasodilators. A type of blood pressure medication that works by relaxing blood vessel walls. Examples include: hydralazine (Apresoline) and minoxidil (Loniten). (For a full discussion of the direct vasodilators see chapter 7.)

Diuretic. One of the first types of medication used in the treatment of high blood pressure. Diuretics are also used to treat heart failure and other heart problems. There are many types of diuretics including thiazides, loop, and potassium-sparing diuretics. Diuretics are generally very inexpensive and are frequently used in combination with other blood pressure medications. Some diuretics can cause elevations in blood cholesterol levels. Diuretics are also known to cause electrolyte disturbances, most notably a loss of potassium. This class of medications is also known to raise blood sugar and uric acid levels. Despite the potential for side effects, low doses of diuretics can almost always be used. (See chapter 7 for a full discussion of diuretics.)

Dubbel Zoote drops. A candy composed of licorice and salt that can cause high blood pressure.

Echocardiogram. A painless procedure that uses sound waves to assess heart muscle and valve function.

Eclampsia. A disorder unique to pregnancy characterized by life-threatening seizures. Generally preceded by preeclampsia.

Edema. Swelling of body tissue due to the buildup of salt and water. In most cases it is the ankles and lower legs that swell.

Electrocardiogram. Often referred to as an EKG or ECG, an electrocardiogram is a painless procedure in which electrodes are placed on the chest wall, arms, and legs and used to monitor electrical impulses as they pass through the heart muscle, controlling its activity. In some situations an EKG is combined with exercise (stress test). This is done to detect electrical disturbances that might not be evident at rest.

Endothelium. The inner lining of an artery.

Ephedrine. A chemical found in many cold medications that can cause high blood pressure.

Erythropoetin. A hormone that stimulates the production of red blood cells, which can also cause high blood pressure.

Fetal alcohol syndrome. Mental retardation occurring in children as a result of *in utero* alcohol exposure.

F.I.T. (frequency/intensity/time) principle. The three things that must be kept in mind as a person develops an exercise program.

Framingham Heart Study. An extremely important heart study performed in Framingham, Massachusetts. This study helped identify many of the heart disease risk factors. Although the original Framingham Heart Study is over, the Framingham Offspring Study continues. The people of Framingham have participated in studies for over fifty years.

Gastric bypass surgery. A procedure used to treat morbid obesity. A small pouch is constructed between the esophagus and the intestines. The stomach is bypassed and the pouch serves as a new and very small stomach.

Genetics. The study of heredity.

Habitrol. See *Nicotine patch.*

Heart attack. See *Myocardial infarction.*

Heart failure. Frequently called "congestive heart failure," this condition occurs when the heart muscle is unable to adequately pump blood from the heart to the rest of the body. People with heart failure often experience fluid buildup in the ankles, feet, and lungs. Heart failure can occur following a heart attack, especially when a large part of the heart muscle has been damaged.

HELLP syndrome. A syndrome occurring in pregnancy consisting of Hemolysis (destruction of red blood cells), Elevated Liver function tests, and Low Platelets. The only definitive therapy is delivery.

High blood pressure. See *Hypertension.*

High-density lipoprotein cholesterol (HDL-C). Often referred to as "the good cholesterol," high levels of this lipoprotein protect against the development of cardiac disease through a process called reverse cholesterol transport.

HMG CoA reductase inhibitor. A class of cholesterol-lowering drugs including atorvastatin (Lipitor), lovastatin (Mevacor), simvastatin (Zocor), cerevastatin (Baycol), pravastatin (Pravachol), and fluvastatin (Lescol).

Hypercholesterolemia. An elevated blood cholesterol level.

Hypercortisolism (Cushing's syndrome). A disorder characterized by the overproduction of cortisol from the adrenal gland. One of the findings in this disorder is high blood pressure.

Hyperparathyroidism. A condition characterized by excess blood levels of parathyroid hormone. It can occur if one of the four parathyroid glands contains a tumor or as a result of diffuse enlargement of all four glands. Signs and symptoms of hyperparathyroidism include high blood pressure and elevated blood calcium levels.

Hypertension. A condition characterized by sustained high blood pressure and an increased risk of heart disease, stroke, and kidney failure. While lifestyle changes such as salt and alcohol restriction, exercise, weight loss, and smoking cessation may normalize blood pressure, there are cases when medications are necessary.

Hypertensive Optimal Treatment (HOT) Study. A study including 19,000 hypertensive people designed to determine the optimal blood pressure goal for people with high blood pressure. Therapy may involve either medications or surgery.

Hyperthyroidism. A condition in which the thyroid gland is overactive. This condition can lead to high blood pressure.

Hypoglycemia. Low blood sugar.

Hypothyroidism. A condition in which the thyroid gland is underactive. This condition can lead to high blood pressure. Therapy involves daily thyroid replacement in the form of a pill.

Insulin. A hormone produced by the pancreas. This hormone promotes the entry of sugar into the cells.

Insulin resistance. A disorder characterized by decreased responsiveness to the hormone insulin. As compared to people without insulin resistance, persons with this disorder must produce significantly larger amounts of insulin to maintain the same blood sugar level.

Ischemia. An imbalance between the oxygen demand of a portion of the heart muscle and the oxygen supply delivered to that portion of the heart muscle. Ischemia is the result of a blockage within one or more of the coronary arteries.

Joint National Committee on Prevention, Detection, Evaluation, and Treatment of High Blood Pressure (JNC). A national committee of experts in the field of high blood pressure who have met periodically since 1988. This committee has published six reports on the prevention, detection, evaluation, and treatment of high blood pressure in the United States, the most recent in 1997.

Kempner's rice diet. In the 1940s this diet consisting mainly of rice was a popular method of blood pressure reduction.

Lescol. A cholesterol-lowering medication.

Lipid. A blood fat. Examples include LDL-cholesterol, HDL-cholesterol, and triglycerides.

Lipitor. A cholesterol-lowering medication.

Lopid. A triglyceride-lowering medication

Low-density lipoprotein cholesterol (LDL-C). Often referred to as "the bad cholesterol," elevated levels of this blood fat increase the risk of developing heart disease.

Lumen. The central channel of a blood vessel through which blood flows.

Magnetic resonance imaging (MRI). A procedure that allows one to view the inner body or brain with the use of a magnetic field. An MRI can often give a clearer picture than can a standard X-ray or CAT (computer-assisted tomography), without exposure to radiation.

Menopause. The time in a woman's life when the ovaries cease to produce the female hormones estrogen and progesterone. In the United States the average woman enters menopause at about age fifty-one. Smokers tend to enter menopause at an earlier age.

Mevacor. A cholesterol-lowering medication.

Monounsaturated fat. The type of fat found in canola oil, olive oil, and peanut oil. This type of fat is also present in avocados and peanuts. When this type of fat is substituted for saturated fat, total cholesterol level will fall and the HDL cholesterol level may rise.

Myocardial infarction. A heart attack. This condition develops when an area of heart muscle is deprived of oxygen. The result is cellular death and eventual scar formation.

National Institutes of Health (NIH). A large governmental organization that performs independent research, conducts national health surveys, produces consensus documents regarding disease states, and provides worthy scientists throughout the United States with research grants.

New England Heart Institute. The largest heart institute in the state of New Hampshire, offering comprehensive cardiac care including cardiac catheterization, angioplasty, intravascular ultrasound, stent placement, electrophysiology, bypass surgery, cardiac rehabilitation, cholesterol management, hypertension therapy, and smoking cessation therapy.

Niaspan. A cholesterol-lowering medication that can lower both LDL-cholesterol and triglycerides while raising HDL-cholesterol.

Nicoderm. See *Nicotine patch.*

Nicotine patch (Habitrol, Nicoderm, Nicotrol, Prostep). Used as a smoking cessation tool, the nicotine patch is placed on the upper arm. Nicotine, the addictive substance found in cigarettes, is delivered from the patch directly into the bloodstream. The dose of the patch is gradually reduced until the user is ready to quit smoking.

Nicotrol. See *Nicotine patch.*

Nonsteroidal anti-inflamatory drugs (NSAIDs). Medications used to treat minor aches and pains as well as chronic conditions such as arthritis. The NSAIDs can also cause high blood pressure by promoting salt and water retention.

Norepinephrine. A stimulant hormone produced by the adrenal gland, also called noradrenaline.

Normotensive. Having normal blood pressure.

Norplant. A long-acting (years) form of birth control consisting of series of five small progesterone implants placed in the subcutaneous tissue of the forearm. The progesterone in the implants gradually seeps into the bloodstream, providing pregnancy protection for up to five years.

Obstructive sleep apnea. A disorder caused by airway obstruction during sleep and characterized by snoring, gasping, and apnea (lack of breathing) during sleep. Sleep apnea is associated with daytime drowsiness and high blood pressure. Therapy typically involves weight loss and alcohol restriction. At times facial appliances are utilized to prevent airway obstruction during sleep. Occasionally surgery will be required.

Orlistat (Xenical). A weight loss medication.

Peripheral sympatholytics. A class of blood pressure–lowering medications that work by blocking the sympathetic nervous system. Examples include: deserpidine (Harmonyl), guanadrel (Hylorel), guanethidine (Ismelin), and reserpine (Serpasil). For a full discussion of peripheral sympatholytics see chapter 7.

Peripheral vascular disease. A disorder characterized by atherosclerosis of the lower extremities. The most common symptom of PVD is claudication or leg pain, which occurs with walking.

Phentermine (Ionamin). A weight loss medication.

Phenylephrine. A chemical found in many cold medications that can cause high blood pressure.

Phenylpropanolamine. A chemical found in many cold medications that can cause high blood pressure.

Pheochromocytoma. An endocrine tumor of the adrenal medulla that secretes hormones either continuously or intermittently. Signs and symptoms of this tumor may include headache, high blood pressure, sweating, palpitations, and a feeling of doom.

Pituitary gland. A small gland found at the base of the brain responsible for the secretion of a number of hormones. These hormones in turn regulate many bodily processes including growth, reproduction, and metabolic activities. Disorders of the pituitary gland can result in many disorders including high blood pressure.

Placebo. An inert medication or sugar pill often used in research trials.

Plaque. A blockage within an artery composed of cholesterol, cellular debris, inflammatory cells, and fibrous material.

Platelet. A blood-clotting cell.

Polyunsaturated fat. The type of fat found in corn, sunflower, and safflower oils. When this type of fat is substituted for saturated fat, both total and HDL-cholesterol levels may fall.

Pravachol. A cholesterol–lowering medication.

Preeclampsia. A condition formerly called "toxemia of pregnancy" characterized by hypertension, headaches, edema in the legs, and protein in the urine. If untreated, life-threatening seizures of eclampsia may occur.

Primary aldosteronism. A disorder caused by a tumor in one of the two adrenal glands or caused by diffuse enlargement of both adrenal glands. One of the major findings in primary aldosteronism is high blood pressure.

Prostep. See *Nicotine patch.*

Protease inhibitors. Drugs used in the therapy of HIV/AIDS.

Pseudoephedrine. A chemical found in many cold medications that can cause high blood pressure.

Pulse. Beating of an artery that can be felt with the fingers and used to determine heart rate. There are many locations on the body where a pulse can be felt; the most common are the carotid (in the neck) and the radial (in the wrist).

Refractory high blood pressure. High blood pressure that has failed to fall below 140/90 mmHg despite lifestyle changes and adequate doses of three blood pressure medications (one of which is a diuretic).

Renal hypertension. High blood pressure caused by underlying kidney disease.

Renin. A chemical made by the kidney involved in the maintenance of blood pressure.

Renovascular hypertension. High blood pressure caused by blockages in the kidney arteries.

Resistance training. Weight training.

Retinoids (Accutane). A medication used in the treatment of cystic acne. This agent can cause liver abnormalities and elevate cholesterol.

Risk factors. Habits or conditions that may increase a person's risk of developing symptomatic heart disease.

Saphenous vein. A leg vein often surgically removed and used during a bypass procedure. It typically connects the aorta to the heart artery, bypassing the blocked area of the heart artery.

Saturated fat. The type of fat found in butter, cheese, whole milk, ice cream, white marbling in meat, palm and coconut oils. This type of fat is known to increase cholesterol levels dramatically.

Secondary aldosteronism. A disorder characterized by diffuse enlargement of both adrenal glands as a result of underlying kidney disease. One of the findings in secondary aldosteronism is high blood pressure.

Secondary hypertension. High blood pressure resulting from an underlying illness or condition. Causes include kidney disease, primary aldosteronism, secondary hyperaldosteronism, hypercortisolism, pheochromocytoma, hyperthyroidism, hypothyroidism, hyperparathyroidism, obstructive sleep apnea, and morbid obesity. For a full discussion of the causes of secondary hypertension see chapter 9.

Sibutramine (Meridia). A weight loss medication.

Sphygmomanometer. A device used to measure blood pressure.

Stress test. See *Electrocardiogram*.

Stroke. Partial or total loss of function of a part of the body due to brain damage resulting from an interruption of blood flow to the brain.

Syndrome X. A dysmetabolic disorder characterized by high blood pressure, insulin resistance (prediabetes), high blood triglycerides, and low HDL-cholesterol (the protective cholesterol). This syndrome dramatically increases the risk of premature heart disease and has both a genetic and an environmental basis.

Systole. The pressure in the body's arteries as blood is being squeezed out of the heart.

Systolic Hypertension in the Elderly Program (SHEP). A blood pressure–lowering trial in the elderly, which concluded that diuretic therapy for high blood pressure could dramatically reduce the risk of stroke in this population.

Target heart rate. The goal heart rate during exercise. In general the target heart rate is between 50 to 85 percent of a person's maximum heart rate. (An easy way to calculate the maximum heart rate is to subtract a person's age from 220.)

Tissue plasminogen activator (TPA). A clot-dissolving agent.

Tricor. A triglyceride-lowering medication.

Triglyceride. One of the blood fats. Triglycerides may be made by the liver or ingested through the diet. An elevated triglyceride level appears to be a strong predictor of developing heart disease, high blood pressure, and diabetes.

Vasoconstrictor. A substance or chemical that causes the arteries to constrict, leading to an increase in blood pressure.

Wellbutrin. See *Bupropion.*

White coat hypertension. High blood pressure that occurs only in the doctor's office or in other stressful situations.

Zocor. A cholesterol-lowering medication.

Zyban. See *Bupropion.*

Bibliography

PART I: HIGH BLOOD PRESSURE—WHAT IS IT?

Chapter 1: Do I Have It?

"Results from the Third National Health and Nutrition Examination Survey," 1988–91. *Hypertension* 25 (1995): 305–313.

"The Sixth Report of the Joint National Committee on Prevention, Detection, Evaluation, and Treatment of High Blood Pressure." *Archives of Internal Medicine* 157 (1997): 2413–2446. NIH Publication No. 98-4080.

Wilson PWF, D'Agostino RB, Levy D, et al. "Prediction of Coronary Heart Disease Using Risk Factor Categories." *Circulation* 97 (1998): 1837–1847.

Chapter 2: What Causes It? And Why Should I Worry?

Cobb S, Rose RM. "Hypertension, Peptic Ulcers and Diabetes in Air Traffic Controllers." *JAMA* 224 (1973): 489–492.

Hinchliffe SA, Lynch MRJ, Sargent PH, et al. "The Effect of Intrauterine Growth Retardation on the Development of Renal Nephrons." *British Journal of Obstetrics and Gynaecology* 99 (1992): 293–301.

Intersalt Cooperative Research Group. "Intersalt: An International Study of Electrolyte Excretion and Blood Pressure. Results for 24-Hour Urinary Sodium and Potassium Excretion." *British Medical Journal* 297 (1988): 319–328.

Kannel WB, Garrison RJ, Dannenberg AL. "Secular Blood Pressure Trends in Normotensive Persons: The Framingham Study." *American Heart Journal* 125 (1993): 1154–1158.

Konje JC, Bell SC, Morton JJ, et al. "Human Fetal Kidney Morphometry During Gestation and the Relationship Between Weight, Kidney Morphometry and Plasma Active Renin Concentration at Birth." *Clinical Science* 91 (1996): 169-175.

Kotchen JM, McKean HE, Kotchen TA. "Blood Pressure Trends with Aging." *Hypertension* 4 (Suppl 3) (1982): III 128-III 134.

Page LB, Vandevert DE, Nader K, et al. "Blood Pressure of Quash' qai Pastoral Nomads in Iran in Relation to Culture, Diet, and Body Form." *American Journal of Clinical Nutrition* 34 (1981): 527-538.

Perini C, Muller FB, Buhler FR. "Suppressed Aggression Accelerates Early Development of Essential Hypertension." *Journal of Hypertension* 9 (1991): 499-503.

Schneider RH, Egan BM, Johnson EH, et al. "Anger and Anxiety in Borderline Hypertension." *Psychosomatic Medicine* 48 (1986): 242-248.

Stamler J, Rose G, Stamler R, et al. "Intersalt Study Findings. Public Health and Medical Care Implications." *Hypertension* 14 (1989): 570-577.

Timio M, Verdecchia P, Venanzi S, et al. "Age and Blood Pressure Changes: A 20-Year Follow-Up Study in Nuns in a Secluded Order." *Hypertension* 12 (1988): 457-461.

PART II: TREATMENT

Chapter 3: Diet and Blood Pressure—The Critical Link

Allender PS, Cutler JA, Follmann D, et al. "Dietary Calcium and Blood Pressure: A Meta-Analysis of Randomized Clinical Trials." *Annals of Internal Medicine* 124 (1996): 825-831.

Appel LJ, Miller III ER, Seidler AJ, et al. "Does Supplementation of Diet with 'Fish Oil' Reduce Blood Pressure?" *Archives of Internal Medicine* 153 (1993): 1429-1438.

Appel LJ, Moore TJ, Obarzanek E, et al. for the DASH Collaborative Research Group. "A Clinical Trial of the Effects of Dietary Patterns on Blood Pressure." *New England Journal of Medicine* 336 (1997): 1117-1124.

Burke V, Beilin L. "Vegetarian Diets and High Blood Pressure: An Update." *Nutrition Metabolism and Cardiovascular Disease* 4 (1994): 103-112.

Kempner W. "Treatment of Hypertensive Vascular Disease with Rice Diet." *American Journal of Medicine* 4 (1948): 545–577.

Morris MC, Sacks F, Rosner B. "Does Fish Oil Lower Blood Pressure? A Meta-Analysis of Controlled Trials." *Circulation* 88 (1993): 523–533.

National Heart, Lung, and Blood Institute. "How to Prevent High Blood Pressure." National Institute of Health Publication No. 96-3281, 1996.

Omvik P, Myking OL. "Unchanged Central Hemodynamics After Six Months of Moderate Sodium Restriction with or Without Potassium Supplementation in Essential Hypertension." *Blood Pressure* 4 (1995): 32–41.

The Sixth Report of the Joint National Committee on Prevention, Detection, Evaluation, and Treatment of High Blood Pressure. *Archives of Internal Medicine* 157 (1997): 2413–2446. National Institute of Health Publication No. 98-4080.

Stamler J, Caggiula A, Grandits GA, et al. "Relationship to Blood Pressure of Combinations of Dietary Macronutrients." Findings of the Multiple Risk Factor Intervention Trial (MRFIT). *Circulation* 94 (1996): 2417–2423.

Ueshima H, Mikawa K, Baba S, et al. "Effect of Reduced Alcohol Consumption on Blood Pressure in Untreated Hypertensive Men." *Hypertension* 21 (1993): 248–252.

Welton PK. "Potassium and Blood Pressure." Izzo JL, Black and HR, eds. *Hypertension Primer: The Essentials of Hypertension.* Dallas: American Heart Association, 1993.

Welton PK, Appel LJ, Espeland MA, et al. for the TONE Collaborative Research Group. "Sodium Reduction and Weight Loss in the Treatment of Hypertension in Older Persons: A Randomized Controlled Trial of Nonpharmacologic Interventions in the Elderly (TONE)." *JAMA* 279 (1998): 839–846.

Welton PK, Klag MJ. "Magnesium and Blood Pressure: Review of the Epidemiologic and Clinical Trial Experience." *American Journal of Cardiology* 63 (1989): 26G–30G.

Chapter 4: Developing an Exercise Program

Bailey C. *The New Fit or Fat*. Boston: Houghton Mifflin, 1991.

Kokkinos PF, Narayan P, Colleran JA, et al. "Effects of Regular Exercise on Blood Pressure and Left Ventricular Hypertrophy in African-American Men with Severe Hypertension." *New England Journal of Medicine* 333 (1995): 1462–1467.

McGowan MP. *Heart Fitness for Life*. New York: Oxford University Press, 1997.

Paffenbarger RS Jr, Hyde RT, Wing AL, et al. "The Association of Changes in Physical-Activity Level and Other Lifestyle Characteristics with Mortality Among Men." *New England Journal of Medicine* 328 (1993): 538–545.

Papademetriou V, Kokkinos PF. "The Role of Exercise in the Control of Hypertension and Cardiovascular Risk." *Current Opinions: Nephrology Hypertension* 5 (1996): 459–462.

Shaper AG, Wannamethee G, Walker M. "Physical Activity, Hypertension and Risk of Heart Attack in Men Without Evidence of Ischaemic Heart Disease." *Journal of Human Hypertension* 8 (1994): 3–10.

U.S. Department of Health and Human Services. "Physical Activity and Health: A Report of the Surgeon General." Atlanta, GA: Centers for Disease Control and Prevention, National Center for Chronic Disease Prevention and Health Promotion, 1996.

Ward A, Taylor PA, Ahlquist L, et al. "Exercise and Exercise Intervention." Ockene IS and Ockene JK, eds. *Prevention of Coronary Heart Disease*. Boston: Little, Brown, 1992.

Chapter 5: Weight Loss

Abenhaim L, Moride Y, Brenot F, et al. "Appetite Suppressant Drugs and the Risk of Primary Pulmonary Hypertension." *New England Journal of Medicine* 335 (1996): 609–616.

Connolly HM, Crary JL, McGoon MD, et al. "Valvular Heart Disease Associated with Fenfluramine-phentermine." *New England Journal of Medicine* 337 (1997): 581–588.

Darne' B, Nivarong M, Tugaye' A, et al. "Hypocaloric Diet and Anti-hypertensive Drug Treatment. A Randomized Controlled Clinical Trial." *Blood Pressure* 2 (1993): 130–135.

"Executive Summary of the Clinical Guidelines on the Identification, Evaluation, and Treatment of Overweight and Obesity in Adults." *Archives of Internal Medicine* 158 (1998): 1855–1867.

Gordon NF, Scott CB, Levine BD. "Comparison on Single versus Multiple Lifestyle Interventions." *American Journal of Cardiology* 79 (1997): 763–767.

Schardt D. "Fat Burners." *Nutrition Action* 26, no. 6 (1999): 9–11.

Chapter 6: You Can Quit Smoking!

Blondal T, Gudmundsson LJ, Olafsdottir I, et al. "Nicotine Nasal Spray with Nicotine Patch for Smoking Cessation: Randomised Trial with-six year follow-up." *British Medical Journal* 318 (1999): 285–289.

Fagerstrom KO. "Measuring Degree of Physical Dependence on Tobacco Smoking with Reference to Individualization of Treatment." *Addictive Behaviors* 3 (1978): 235–241.

Fiore MC, Smith SS, Jorenby DE, et al. "The Effectiveness of the Nicotine Patch for Smoking Cessation." *JAMA* 271 (1994): 1940–1947.

Jorenby DE, Leischow SJ. "A Controlled Trial of Sustained-Release Bupropion, a Nicotine Patch, or Both for Smoking Cessation." *New England Journal of Medicine* 340 (1999): 685–691.

Mann SJ, James GD, Wang RS, Pickering TG. "Elevation of Ambulatory Systolic Blood Pressure in Hypertensive Smokers. A Case Control Study." *JAMA* 265 (1991): 2226–2228.

Okene JK. "Smoking Interventions: A Behavioral, Educational, and Pharmacological Perspective." Ockene IS and Ockene JK, eds. *Prevention of Coronary Heart Disease*. Boston: Little, Brown, 1992.

Verecchia P, Schillaci G, Borgioni C, et al. "Cigarette Smoking, Ambulatory Blood Pressure and Cardiac Hypertrophy in Essential Hypertension." *Journal of Hypertension* 13 (1995): 1209–1215.

Chapter 7: An Overview of Blood Pressure Medications

Abernathy DR. "Pharmacological Properties of Combination Therapies for Hypertension." *American Journal of Hypertension* 10 (1997): 13S–16S.

Acker CG, Greenberg A. "Angioedema Induced by the Angiotensin II Blocker Losartan (Letter)."*New England Journal of Medicine* 333 (1995): 1572.

Alderman MH. "Which Antihypertensive Drugs First—And Why!" *JAMA* 267 (1992): 2786–2787

"The Antihypertensive and Lipid Lowering Treatment to Prevent Heart Attack Trial (ALLHAT)." *JAMA* 283 (2000): 1967–1975.

Cohen HJ, Pieper CF, Hanlon JT, et al. "Calcium Channel Blockers and Cancer." *American Journal of Medicine* 108 (2000): 210–215.

Dahlof B, Linddholm L, Hansson L, et al. "Morbidity and Mortality in the Swedish Trial in Old Patients with Hypertension (STOP-Hypertension)." *Lancet* 338 (1991): 1281–1285.

De Leeuw PW. "How Do Angiotensin II Receptor Antagonists Affect Blood Pressure?" *American Journal of Cardiology* 84 (1999): 5K–6K.

Furberg CD, Psaty BM, Meyer JV. "Nifedipine Dose-Related Increase in Mortality in Patients with Coronary Heart Disease." *Circulation* 92 (1995): 1326–1331.

Gueyffier F, Boutitie F, Boissel JP, et al., for the INDANA Investigators. "Effect of Antihypertensive Drug Treatment on Cardiovascular Outcomes in Women and Men: A Meta-Analysis of Individual Patient Data for Randomized, Controlled Trials." *Annals of Internal Medicine* 126 (1997): 761–767.

Hansson L, Zanchetti A, Carruthers SG, et al. "Effects of Intensive Blood-Pressure Lowering and Low-Dose Aspirin in Patients with Hypertension: Principal Results of the Hypertension Optimal Treatment (HOT) Randomised Trial. HOT Study Group." *Lancet* 351 (1998): 1755–1762.

The Heart Outcomes Prevention Evaluation Study Investigators. "Effects of an Angiotensin–Converting–Enzyme Inhibitor, Ramipril, on Death from Cardiovascular Causes, Myocardial Infarction, and Stroke in High Risk Patients." *New England Journal of Medicine* 342 (2000): 145– 153.

Kaplan NM. *Clinical Hypertension.* Baltimore: Williams & Wilkins, 1998.

Kaplan NM. "Do Calcium Antagonists Cause Myocaardial Infarction?" (editorial). *American Journal of Cardiology* 77 (1996): 81–82.

Levy D, Walmsley P, Levenstein M, for the Hypertension and Lipid Trial Study Group. "Principal Results of the Hypertension and Lipid Trial (HALT): A Multicenter Study of Doxazosin in Patients with Hypertension." *American Heart Journal* 131 (1996): 966–973.

Maggioni AP, Latini R. "How to Use ACE-Inhibitors, Beta-Blockers, and Newer Therapies in AMI." *American Heart Journal* 138 (1999): 183– 187.

Materson BJ, Reda DJ, Cushman WC, et al., for the Department of Veterans Affairs Cooperative Study Group on Antihypertensive Agents. "Single-Drug Therapy for Hypertension in Men: A Comparison of Six Antihypertensive Agents with Placebo." *New England Journal of Medicine* 328 (1993): 914–921.

Messerli FH. "Safety of Calcium Antagonists: Dissecting the Evidence." *American Journal of Cardiology* 78 (Suppl 9A) (1996): 19–23.

Moser M, Pickering T, Sowers JR. "Combination Drug Therapy in the Management of Hypertension: When, With What, and How." *Journal of Clinical Hypertension* 2 (2000): 94–98.

Saseen JJ, Carter BL, Brown TER, et al. "Comparison of Nifedipine Alone with Diltiazem or Verapamil in Hypertension." *Hypertension* 28 (1996): 209–2114.

Soriano JB, Hoes AW, Meems L, et al. "Increased Survival with Beta-Blockers: Importance of Ancillary Properties." *Properties in Cardiovascular Disease* 39 (1997): 445–456.

"The Sixth Report of the Joint National Committee on Prevention, Detection, Evaluation, and Treatment of High Blood Pressure." *Archives of Internal Medicine* 157 (1997): 2413–2446. National Institutes of Health Publication No. 98-4080.

Systolic Hypertension in the Elderly Program Cooperative Research Group. "Implications of the Systolic Hypertension in the Elderly Program." *Hypertension* 21 (1993): 335–343.

Waeber B. "Vasopeptidase Inhibition: A New Approach to the Management of Cardiovascular Disease." *Journal of Clinical Hypertension* 2 (2000): 87–93.

Weir MR. "The Role of Multiple Drug Therapy for Controlling Hypertension in African Americans." *Journal of Clinical Hypertension* 2 (2000): 99–108.

Chapter 8: Home Blood Pressure Monitors

Appel LJ, Stason WB. "Ambulatory Blood Pressure Monitoring and Blood Pressure Self-Measurement in the Diagnosis and Management of Hypertension." *Annals of Internal Medicine* 118 (1993): 867–882.

Ashida T, Sugiyama T, Okuno S, et al. "Relationship Between Home Blood Pressure Measurement and Medication Compliance and Name Recognition of Antihypertensive Drugs." *Hypertension Research* 23 (2000): 21–24.

"Blood-Pressure Monitors: Convenience Doesn't Equal Accuracy." *Consumer Reports* 61, no. 50 (1996): 53–55.

Clark LA, Denby L, Pregibon D, et al. "A Quantitative Analysis of the Effects of Activity and Time of Day on the Diurnal Variations of Blood Pressure." *Journal of Chronic Disease* 40 (1987): 671–679.

Graves JW, Sheps SG. "Out-of-Office Self-Measurement of Blood Pressure." *Journal of Clinical Hypertension* 1 (1999): 120–124.

PART III: MANAGING HYPERTENSION IN SPECIAL SITUATIONS

Chapter 9: When Nothing Seems to Work

Bravo EL. "Management of Hypercortisolism and Hyperaldosteronism." Izzo JL and Black HR, eds. *Hypertension Primer.* Dallas: American Heart Association, 1999.

Ganguly A. "Primary Aldosteronism." *New England Journal of Medicine* 339 (1998): 368–369.

Kaplan NM. *Clinical Hypertension.* Baltimore: Williams & Wilkins, 1998.

Levinson PD, Millman RP. "Management of Sleep Apnea Hypertension." Izzo JL and Black HR, eds. *Hypertension Primer.* Dallas: American Heart Association, 1999.

Nally JV. "Management of Renovascular Hypertension." Izzo JL and Black HR, eds. *Hypertension Primer.* Dallas: American Heart Association, 1999.

Neumann HP, Berger DP, Sigmond G. "Pheochromocytomas, Multiple Endocrine Neoplasia Type 2 and von Hippel-Lindau Disease." *New England Journal of Medicine* 329 (1993): 1531.

Wofford MR, King DS, Wyatt SB, et al. "Secondary Hypertension: Detection and Management for the Primary Care Provider." *Journal of Clinical Hypertension* 2 (2000): 124–131.

Young WF. "Management of Thyroid and Parathyroid Disorders." Izzo JL and Black HR, eds. *Hypertension Primer*. Dallas: American Heart Association, 1999.

Young WF, Sheldon SG. "Management of Pheochromocytoma." Izzo JL and Black HR, eds. *Hypertension Primer*. Dallas: American Heart Association, 1999.

Chapter 10: Hypertension in Special Populations

August P. Preeclampsia: "New Thoughts on an Ancient Problem." *Journal of Clinical Hypertension* 2 (2000): 115–123.

Glorioso N, Troffa C, Filigheddu F, et al. "Effect of the HMG-CoA Reductase Inhibitors on Blood Pressure in Patients with Essential Hypertension and Primary Hypercholesterolemia." *Hypertension* 34 (1999): 1281–1286.

Grimm RH, Flack JM, Granditis GA, et al., for the Treatment of Mild Hypertension Study (TOMHS) Research Group. "Long-Term Effects on Plasma Lipids of Diet and Drugs to Treat Hypertension." *JAMA* 275 (1996): 1549–1556.

Haffner SM, Lehto S, Ronnemaa T, et al. "Mortality for Coronary Heart Disease in Subjects with Type 2 Diabetes and in Nondiabetic Subjects With and Without Prior Myocardial Infarction." *New England Journal of Medicine* 329 (1998): 229–234.

Prisant LM, Moser M. "Hypertension in the Elderly: Can We Improve Results of Therapy?" *Archives of Internal Medicine* 160 (2000): 283–289.

Reaven GM. *Syndrome X: Overcoming the Silent Killer That Can Give You a Heart Attack*. New York: Simon & Schuster, 2000.

Reaven GM, Lithell H, Landsberg L. "Hypertension and Associated Abnormalities—The Role of Insulin Resistance and the Sympathoadrenal System." *New England Journal of Medicine* 334 (1996): 374–381.

Sadowski R, Falkner B. "Evaluation of Hypertension in Older Children and Adolescents." *Journal of Clincial Hypertension* 1 (1999): 125–135.

UK Prospective Diabetes Study Group. "Efficacy of Atenolol and Captopril in Reducing Risk of Macrovascular and Microvascular Complications in Type 2 Diabetes." *United Kingdom Prospective Diabetes Study* 39, 317 (1998): 713–720.

Resources

American Heart Association
1615 Stemmons Freeway
Dallas, TX 75207
800-AHA-USA1
www.americanheart.org

The DASH Diet
http://dash.bwh.harvard

International Society on Hypertension in Blacks
2045 Manchester St. NE
Atlanta, GA 30324
404-875-6263
www.ishib.org

National Heart, Lung, and Blood Institute
P.O. Box 30105
Bethesda, MD 20824
301-592-8573
www.nhlbi.nih.gov.nhlbi.htm

National Hypertension Association
324 East 30th St.
New York, NY 10016
212-889-3557

National Hypertension Hotline
(run by the NHLBI)
800-575-WELL

Index

৯১

ABPM, 161–64
Accutane, 216, 217
acebutolol, 216
ACE inhibitors, 16–17, 18,
   133–39
Adalat, 123, 125, 126, 205
adolescents, 230–35
adrenal ademona, 187
adrenal glands, 184–85
   Cushing's syndrome, 189–92
   11-alpha hydroxylase, 192
   pheochromocytoma, 192–96
   primary aldosteronism, 182–88
   secondary hyperaldosteronism,
      188
   17-beta hydroxylase, 192
adrenaline, 18
adrenocorticotropic hormone
   (ACTH), 189–90
aerobic exercise, 58, 59. See also exercise
African Americans, 3
   ACE inhibitors, 137
   beta-blockers, 114–15

children, 231
DASH Trial participants, 34
diuretics, 99, 104
diuretics, use of, 104
salt intake, 15
sartans, 140
sodium reduction, 47
age and aging, 3, 15, 19–20.
   See also elderly people
Agenrase capsules, 216
AIDS patients, 217
air traffic controllers, 19
alcohol consumption, 3, 23–24, 54,
   161, 168, 169, 199
Aldomet, 149
aldosteronism, primary, 182–88
alpha-adrenergic blockers, 142–45
alpha-beta-receptor antagonists,
   145–48
Altace, 206, 237
Alzheimer's disease, 131
ambulatory blood pressure
   monitoring (ABPM), 161–64
Amiodorone, 215

271

norepinephrine, 142, 151, 193
Normodyne, 116, 145
Norplant, 26
Norvasc, 102, 118, 121, 123, 125, 126, 127, 131, 132, 206, 207, 237
Norvir, 216
NSAIDs (nonsteroidal anti-inflammatory drugs), 28
Nuprin, 237

obsesity. *See* overweight people
older people. *See* elderly people
orange juice, 125
organ transplant patients, 28
orlistat, 76, 78–80
Ortho Tri-Cyclen, 216
osteoporosis, 189, 237
"overnight 1 milligram dexamethasone suppression test," 190
overweight people, 3, 20–23, 70
  children, 233
  Cushing's syndrome, 189
  morbid obsesity, 199–202

Pacerone, 215
penbutolol, 216
peripheral sympatolytics, 148–49, 151–52
peripheral vascular disease (PVD), 223–25
phentermine, 76, 77
phenylephrine, 27
phenylpropanolamine, 27

pheochromocytoma, 192–96
pindolol, 216
pituitary tumors, 189–90, 191
placebo group studies, 29
Plendil, 123, 125
polycystic kidney disease, 173
potassium, 34, 36, 39
potassium-sparing diuretics, 106, 111–12
PPH, 77
Pravachol, 214, 223
prazosin, 143, 144
preclampsia, 225–28
predictors, 24–25
prednisone, 27, 216, 217
pregnancy, 225–30
primary aldosteronism, 182–88
Procardia, 123, 125, 126, 205
progestin implants, 26
progestin-only pills, 26
progestins, 216, 217
Prometrium, 216
propranolol, 112, 116, 117, 127, 206, 216
prostate enlargement, 143
Prostep, 90
protease inhibitors, 217
protein restriction, 170
Provera, 216
pseudoephedrine, 27
pulmonary hypertension (PPH), 77
pulse rate, checking, 60–61
PVD, 223–25
pyruvate, 81

smoking
blood pressure and, 83–84, 161, 168
HDL cholesterol and, 215
pheochromocytoma "spells," 193
quitting, 83–95
sodium. *See* salt/sodium
"spells" (pheochromocytoma), 193–94
sphygmomanometer, 5
steroids, 27
aldosterone, 185
angioedema, 138
diuretics and, 107
high cholesterol and, 217–18
triglycerides and cholesterol, 216
STOP-1, 236
stress, 18–19, 115
stress test, 5, 204
stretch marks, 189
strokes, 219–23
surgery
adrenal tumor, 192
endocrine tumors, 195–96
gastric bypass surgery, 200, 201
parathyroid gland, 198
pituitary microsurgery, 191–92
renal artery bypass surgery, 178
uvulopalatopharyngoplasty, 199
sweating, excess, 197
Swedish Trial in Old Patients with Hypertension (STOP-1), 236
sympathomimetic amines, 27

sympatolytics
central sympatolytics, 148–51
peripheral sympatolytics, 148–49, 151–52
Syndrome X, 23, 207–12
systolic blood pressure, 5–6, 15, 19–20, 159, 238
Systolic Hypertension in Europe (SYST-EUR) Study, 219, 236
Systolic Hypertension in the Elderly Program (SHEP), 102, 219, 236

"Talk Test," 62
target heart rate (THR), 61–62
improvement exercise stage, 66
initial conditioning, 63, 64
maintenance exercise stage, 67
Tenormin, 114, 116, 117, 118, 206, 216
terazosin, 143, 144
Testoderm, 215
thiazide-related compounds, 105
thiazides, 105
thirst, excessive, 198
Tiazec, 206
Timolide, 117, 118
tissue plasminogen activator (TPA), 221
Toprol, 113, 114, 116, 117, 206, 216
torsemide, 105, 172
Trandate, 145
trandolapril, 102, 135